THE BLOOD PRESSURE BOOK

THE BLOOD PRESSURE BOOK
How to Get It Down and Keep It Down

Stephen P. Fortmann, M.D.
Prudence E. Breitrose, M.A.

STANFORD CENTER FOR RESEARCH
IN DISEASE PREVENTION

BULL PUBLISHING COMPANY
Palo Alto, California

Library of Congress Cataloging-in-Publication Data

Fortmann, Stephen P.
  The blood pressure book: how to get it down and keep it down/
Stephen P. Fortmann, Prudence E. Breitrose.
    p. cm.
  Includes index.
  ISBN 0-923521-32-1 (alk. paper)
  1. Hypertension—Popular works. I. Breitrose, Prudence E.
II. Title.
RC685.H8F624   1995
616. 1' 32—dc20   95-11231
                                                    CIP

Manufactured in the United States of America
10 9 8 7 6 5 4 3 2 1

Bull Publishing Company
P. O. Box 208
Palo Alto, CA 94302

Publisher, James Bull; *production editor,* Julianna Scott Fein; *manuscript editor,* Margaret Moore; *designer and art editor,* Susan Breitbard; *illustrator,* Joan Carol. The text was set in 11.5/13 Adobe Garamond by Thompson Type and printed on 50# White Husky Offset Smooth by Diversified Printing and Publishing Services, Inc.

Acknowledgments

The authors would like to acknowledge the contribution of the Stanford Center for Research in Disease Prevention, whose research staff developed self-help behavior change programs on which some of the sections of this book are modeled.

Foreword

What does it take to make people with high blood pressure do something about it?

Although millions of those with high blood pressure *are* taking care of their problem, and can expect longer, healthier lives as a result, millions are not. It is estimated that of the sixty million people in this country whose pressure is too high, half have not managed to get it under control (or, in many cases, have not even tried). As a result, they are running a risk of stroke and heart disease that is much higher than it need be. And that's tragic. Compared to other life-threatening conditions, high blood pressure is one of the simplest problems to treat; in virtually all cases, pressure can be brought down to safer levels, often without medication.

So why don't people bring their pressure down? One reason is that many of them don't even know they have it, because there are usually no symptoms. But millions *do* know they have high blood pressure—and are *still* not taking those relatively simple steps that could solve their problem for good.

As many physicians know all too well, just telling patients what they should do for their health is unlikely to be effective. And that is why we welcome approaches of the type offered by this book. Rather than simply informing people of their risks, and of the measures they should take, the book leads its readers into action. It enables them to develop their own custom-made blood pressure control program, step by step.

First, the book encourages readers to use the medical system to their advantage, working with doctors to find the right medication if one is needed. Then it leads them into a personalized program to change those elements in their daily routine that may be raising their blood pressure, whether they need to control weight, cut down on sodium, get more exercise, reduce stress—or all of the above. In all cases, readers are aided by quizzes and self-assessments that enable them to find an appropriate starting point for change, and measure their progress.

In the 1970s and 1980s, something wonderful happened: The epidemic of heart disease that had been scorching this country began to decline, and the rate of strokes fell even more sharply. Why? Partly it was because of greater awareness of the need for changes in diet and exercise habits. Partly, it was due to the reduction in cigarette smoking that occurred in those years. But partly—particularly where stroke was concerned—it was due to better control of blood pressure.

Now, however, there are signs that the rate of stroke may be climbing up again. And that may well be due to the fact that blood pressures are inching back up. But if you are one of those now at risk, there is absolutely no reason why you should put up with that risk for a moment longer.

High blood pressure is not a mystery. Its treatment is one of the success stories of medical science. There is only one problem—the patient has to choose to be part of that success story. If that's your choice, as you will see from this book, your high blood pressure could soon be a thing of the past.

Dr. Stephen Fortmann and Prudence Breitrose have long been part of the research and educational team of the Stanford Center for Research in Disease Prevention, and have been major contributors to the Center's goal of putting science into action.

Dr. Fortmann, now Deputy Director of the Center, has conducted research into methods of treating high blood pressure without drugs, and sees many patients with high blood pressure at the Stanford University School of Medicine, where he is Director of the Preventive Cardiology Clinic. Ms. Breitrose has been the major force in creating the educational materials that give the public the ideas, motivation and skills to attack their health problems—including high blood pressure. This work is an excellent example of teamwork between science and communication, and it can have a great impact on all who read it and follow its guidelines.

John W. Farquhar, M.D.
Professor of Medicine, Stanford University School of Medicine
Director, Stanford Center for Research in Disease Prevention

Contents

Introduction

This book is for people who are concerned about high blood pressure for one of these reasons:

- They already have it;
- Or their pressure is showing signs of going up, and they want to get it back under control;
- Or they have high blood pressure in the family, and don't want family history to repeat itself;
- Or they simply want to avoid it.

ABOUT THIS BOOK

In addition to giving you basic information about the causes and treatment of high blood pressure, the book provides a number of "checkups" that will help you find out where you stand, and lead you to practical advice that is tailored to your own needs. This advice is broken down into a series of small steps that individually are easy to take. By the end of the book, the small changes should have added up to a way of living that will help

1

get your pressure down (or keep it from going up) and also improve your general health.

There are three main parts.

Part 1: What's Going On?

- Understanding your pressure
- Working with your doctor
- Understanding and taking medication (if you need it)

Part 2: What Changes Do You Need to Make?

- Assessing your own main needs
- Planning for changes

Part 3: Change Sections

Section 1: Sodium

- How sodium affects blood pressure
- Finding out what foods are high in sodium
- Learning to live with less sodium

Section 2: Weight

- How weight affects blood pressure
- How to bring your weight down without starving yourself

Section 3: Exercise

- How physical activity can make a difference
- How to get started on a walking program
- Other exercise options

Section 4: Stress

- What stress does to blood pressure
- Identifying the causes of stress in your life
- What you can do to reduce (or live with) stress

Section 5: Fine-tuning Your Life

- Things to think about: alcohol, caffeine, and nicotine

Part 1

What's Going On?

This is the way blood pressure is *supposed* to work:

As your heart pushes blood through the arteries, the blood is constantly under pressure, much as water in a garden hose is under pressure when you turn it on. The pressure changes hundreds of times a day as different parts of the body make new demands for the oxygen and nutrients carried in the blood. The heart may pump harder, and the blood vessels expand or contract to direct blood to the parts of the body that need it.

For example, if your legs are working hard to carry you up a hill, pressure will rise as your heart beats more strongly to supply that oxygen. The same thing can happen if you are under stress and your body prepares itself for action. When you calm down or stop exercising—if all is well—pressure returns to normal.

Unfortunately, it doesn't always work this way. If you have high blood pressure, or **hypertension** as it is called, the pressure stays up all the time at a level that is higher than it should be. That means the little arteries in your body are not opening wide enough to let the blood flow through them freely. As a result, blood backs up, and there's pressure all the way back to your heart. The pressure pushes hard against the walls of the arteries, much as water will push against the walls of a garden hose if you partially cover

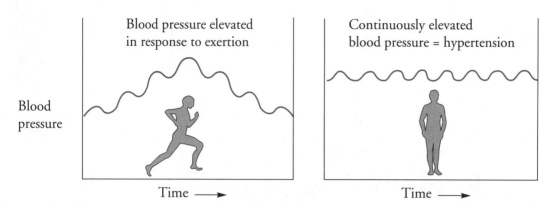

| Blood pressure elevated in response to exertion | Continuously elevated blood pressure = hypertension |

Healthy blood pressure goes up when you are exercising or if you are excited about something, but then it comes down again. When you have high blood pressure, it stays up most of the time.

the end of it with your thumb. And this can cause damage, as you will see on page 5.

WHAT KEEPS PRESSURE TOO HIGH?

In a very few cases, high blood pressure is caused by a specific condition such as kidney disease. But in the great majority of cases, the problem lies with the complex regulation system for blood pressure itself. When all goes well, the blood-pressure control system is set to maintain a certain pressure—much like a thermostat that's set to maintain a certain room temperature. In people with high blood pressure, the base level is simply set too high. All components of the control system work to maintain that high pressure, by narrowing the vessels through which the blood flows, retaining too much fluid and sodium in the blood, and so on.

Looking for Causes

If your blood pressure stays up all the time, and it is not being affected by some other disease, your condition is called **primary hypertension.** "Primary," in this case, means that there's no *other* disease making your blood pressure go up. "Hypertension" means that the tension in the arteries is high. (Primary hypertension is sometimes called *essential hypertension*, but this is a misleading term.)

Doctors don't know precisely *why* one person develops hypertension while someone with exactly the same living and eating habits keeps a healthy pressure for life. But they do know which factors make it much more likely that pressure will rise and stay up:

Factor 1: Family   A tendency to get high blood pressure can be inherited (even though not all people in the same family will necessarily develop it).

Factor 2: Race   For some reason, African Americans are much more likely to develop high blood pressure than Caucasians (even though not all African Americans are at risk).

Factor 3: Mineral Balance   You are more likely to get high blood pressure if you eat a high-sodium, low-potassium diet (even though many people who eat a lot of sodium get lucky and have pressure that stays low for life).

Factor 4: Overweight   Pressure is often closely linked to excess weight (even though some overweight people have pressure that is beautifully low).

WHAT HIGH PRESSURE DOES TO YOU

When there is increased pressure in your arteries, day after day, month after month, it causes wear and tear on the artery walls. This can hurt you in a number of ways:

- Where the artery walls are damaged, cholesterol and other material can get caught in the rough spots and build up to a point where arteries can be blocked. If this happens in the coronary arteries that supply blood to the heart muscle, the result is a heart attack. If it happens in an artery supplying blood to the brain, the result is a stroke.
- Sometimes the pressure can weaken an artery wall to the point where it may burst. This causes a stroke if it happens in the brain, or massive bleeding elsewhere.
- Over the years, high blood pressure can damage the heart, leading to heart failure; or the eyes, leading to blindness; or the kidneys, leading to kidney failure and the need for dialysis treatment.

High blood pressure is especially serious for people who have high levels of cholesterol in their blood.

Why? Excess cholesterol in the blood will form **plaque** at the places where arteries are damaged by the high blood pressure. This will mean a much higher risk that the artery will become totally blocked, leading to a heart attack or a stroke.

High blood pressure is especially damaging for people who smoke.

Why? Tobacco smoke damages the artery walls. If high blood pressure is also tearing away at them, the arteries get double the injury.

High blood pressure is especially damaging for women taking birth control pills.

Why? There's an increased tendency for blood clots to form when you are taking birth control pills, and these can block arteries damaged by constant high pressure.

Some Numbers

On its own, high blood pressure can increase your risk of a heart attack by three to four times, and it can make a stroke more than four times as likely. If you are also a smoker, or have high blood cholesterol, the combination can make your risk very high indeed.

All of that would be quite alarming if you couldn't do anything about high blood pressure—but you can. So before you feel sorry for yourself, consider these two facts:

1. By the time you have worked through this book, not only will you have reduced your blood pressure (or your risk of getting high blood pressure) but you also may have cut the risk of getting other diseases, including heart disease and some types of cancer. And you will do more than just avoid disease—you should end up with more energy and pleasure in living than before you made the changes suggested in this book.

2. If you have been diagnosed as having high blood pressure (or pressure that is on the way up), you are much better off than the millions of Americans who have high blood pressure and don't even know it! It's estimated that of the 60 million or more people in this country who have high pressure, as many as 30–50% may be unaware of their

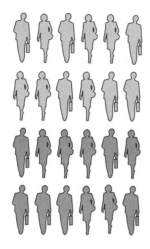

As many as half of the more than sixty million Americans with high blood pressure are unaware of their condition.

problem—**because there are usually no symptoms.** Those people may continue to run a high risk of developing health problems. You, on the other hand, can do a lot to cut those risks—starting now.

MEASURING BLOOD PRESSURE

There are usually no symptoms of high blood pressure, even when pressure is dangerously high. That's why it is important to have your pressure measured regularly, or to measure it yourself.

Throughout this book there are "checkups" that will help you find out your current status. The first checkup concerns your knowledge of your own pressure. If you cannot complete this checkup now, come back to it when you know your pressure.

YOUR PRESSURE   Checkup No. 1

If you know your pressure, write the numbers here:

High number (systolic):   _____

Low number (diastolic):   _____

Date: _____

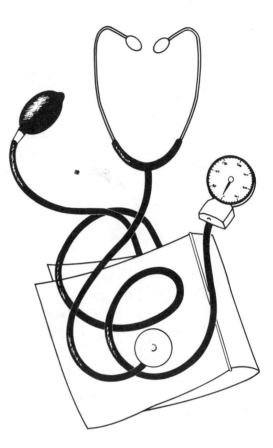

Getting your pressure measured (or measuring your own) is painless—it's just a little squeeze.

How your pressure was measured (check one)

____ Doctor or nurse

____ Automatic coin-operated machine

____ Your own equipment

____ Someone else's equipment

____ Other _____

How Pressure Is Measured

Getting your blood pressure checked is one of the simplest tests you can have, as well as one of the most important. It is also painless.

There are many devices for measuring blood pressure, but they all use basically the same system:

1. A cuff squeezes your upper arm until the blood flow through the main artery in the arm is briefly cut off.
2. As the pressure is gradually released, the machine (or someone with a stethoscope, listening to sounds) can tell at what point blood starts to flow through the artery again. This is the moment when the pressure in the artery is stronger than the pressure in the cuff. That's the high number (systolic) giving the pressure when the heart is actually beating (contracting).
3. As the pressure in the cuff continues to go down, the machine (or the person with the stethoscope) can pick up the point where the pressure in the artery is equal to the pressure in the cuff between heartbeats. That's the low number (diastolic), giving the pressure between contractions.

The Blood Pressure Range

Here are the blood pressure numbers for "ideal," "normal," "borderline," and "high":

	Systolic	Diastolic
Ideal	Under 120	Under 80
Normal	120–129	80–84
Borderline (high normal)	130–140	85–90
High	Over 140	Over 90

Sometimes people have an excellent systolic but a high diastolic, or the other way around. This needs attention, just as it would if both numbers were high, because each number is important.

You may have heard that blood pressure goes up with age—and in America that is usually true. But it doesn't have to. In societies where people live in the way suggested in this book, people's pressure at age 55 is more or less what it was at 20. That's one good reason why everyone in the family should consider taking measures to control pressure, even if it is not high yet.

Trusting the Numbers

Blood pressure goes up and down according to what you are doing. For example, it will go up if you are excited or when you are exercising, and it will go down again when you are relaxed. The numbers may also vary according to the equipment or to the skill of the person using it.

Here are some questions to help you decide if your most recent blood pressure reading was reliable:

Was your pressure measured by someone who knew what he or she was doing?

Doctors, nurses, paramedics, and other health professionals know what they are doing. Your neighbor, trying out his new blood pressure kit, may not.

Was the equipment reliable?

Equipment used in doctors' offices, clinics, or screenings can be trusted. So can some (but not all) of the coin-operated machines available for public use in stores. Not all do-it-yourself devices are as reliable (see page 15 for purchasing suggestions).

Were you calm?

Stress, excitement, and physical activity can all boost blood pressure temporarily. So can coffee, if you are not used to it. You need to sit quietly for a while before the test to get a valid measurement—and don't talk while it is going on.

Was your pressure measured more than once?

Even with the best measurement techniques, blood pressure can change from moment to moment. It is best to average at least three readings, preferably on different days—and, if possible, at different times of day.

White Coat Hypertension

Sometimes blood pressure goes up at the sight of a white coat—in other words, in the doctor's office. Some studies have shown that *most* people with high blood pressure show a slight rise in pressure in the presence of a doctor. In some cases, the rise is quite steep.

In the doctor's office, this effect can be reduced if you sit quietly for a while before your blood pressure is measured. It may be helpful to take a few deep breaths before the test. And don't talk while it is going on.

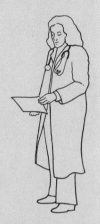

If you and your doctor feel that you cannot get a true reading when there are white coats around, he or she may suggest other ways to get your blood pressure measured. The more readings you can get to make your average, the better. You might be able to benefit from a reliable home system (see page 15). Or your doctor could provide you with an ambulatory system—one that you carry with you to monitor your pressure throughout the day. This can also be helpful in alerting you to other circumstances in your daily routine that cause your pressure to rise.

You won't be able to skip measurements in the doctor's office completely, because those are the numbers that form the basis of what we know about high blood pressure. So talk to your doctor about ways to cut down on your level of tension. (Maybe he or she could take off the white coat!)

Sometimes the mere sight of a white coat can send pressure up.

TRANSLATING THE NUMBERS

If Your Pressure Is "Ideal"   If your pressure is in the ideal range (120/80 or below), this book will help you keep it that way.

If Your Pressure Is "Normal"   Doctors may tell you that pressure between 120/80 and 130/85 is "normal," because it's usual for pressure to edge up into this range in American adults. That doesn't mean it's great—in fact, if your pressure used to be really low, having it edge up into the "normal" zone could be a sign that it is going up, and that you should take steps to keep it from going any higher.

If Your Pressure Is "Borderline"   A reading between 130/85 and 140/90 does not yet mean "hypertension"—but you could be on your way. You should certainly monitor your pressure carefully, getting it checked at least once a year. You should also take measures to get it back where it belongs (in other words, follow the advice in this book).

If Your Pressure Is "High"   When pressure is high (over 140/90) it needs attention. If it's not much above 140/90, it can probably be treated without medication, but you need to make that decision with your doctor. Whether you get medication or not (see page 17 for more on that), your pressure should definitely be brought down.

- Any high pressure can increase your risk of heart attacks and strokes.
- Once your pressure has started going up, there is a good chance it will keep on rising, and you could be in more trouble within a few years.

WORKING WITH THE DOCTOR

It may be that your high pressure was detected at a routine medical visit, in which case your doctor will know about it. But if you pick it up in some other way (for example, on a coin-operated machine) and if your pressure is borderline or above, you should make an appointment to discuss it with a doctor.

Communicating with the Doctor

Here are some tips to help you make the most of your time with the doctor:

- Before the appointment, make notes about any questions you want to ask.
- Make sure you understand everything the doctor tells you. If something is not clear, ask him or her to repeat it.
- Make notes of instructions, or ask the doctor to write them down or give you printed information.

- Before you leave, make sure you know when you should make another appointment, and what you should do before then.
- If you find that your doctor doesn't answer your questions, and can't explain things in a way that satisfies you, consider switching to another doctor. You may be treating blood pressure for life, and it's important to feel from the beginning that you and the doctor understand each other.

The Examination

If your blood pressure is higher than it should be, the doctor will want to examine you carefully to decide how serious the problem is. As part of the examination, he or she will probably do the following:

- Measure your pressure in both arms, standing and sitting
- Ask questions about the health of your parents, brothers, and sisters
- Check your weight and height
- Take a urine sample to check on your kidneys
- Ask how much sodium you take in, especially in the form of salt
- Ask about your alcohol and caffeine intake, exercise habits, and stress
- Ask about other drugs you are taking, such as birth control pills, decongestants, and even street drugs
- Ask you questions about other health habits that could make high blood pressure more dangerous, such as smoking or eating a high-fat diet.

The doctor may arrange for blood tests to check your cholesterol and potassium levels, and other tests as needed.

Your Cholesterol

Knowing your cholesterol level can be important. High levels combined with high blood pressure can greatly increase the risk of heart attack. Here are some numbers to show where cholesterol levels should be:

	Total cholesterol
Ideal	180 or below
OK	180–200
Borderline	200–240
High	Over 240

If your blood pressure is quite high, or if your total cholesterol itself is on the high side, then your doctor may decide to check the *type* of cholesterol in your blood. That's because not all cholesterol is harmful: There's a "good" type that can help your body get rid of the "bad" types.

The type of cholesterol that's helpful is called HDL (high-density lipoprotein). Your aim should be to increase the proportion of HDL, while reducing the other types of cholesterol. Here are the HDL figures to aim for:

	HDL cholesterol
Too low	Under 35
Medium	36–50
Good	Over 50

NOTE: Some tests report only total cholesterol. So *before* you have the blood test for cholesterol, tell your doctor you'd like to know the HDL number.

Adjusting Cholesterol Levels

Although this book is aimed at reducing high blood pressure, it will also give you a healthier cholesterol profile. If your total cholesterol is very high, your doctor may suggest special measures, including drugs, to bring it down. Whether or not you are given drugs, you should reduce the fats in your diet (see page 61), lose weight (page 53), and get more regular exercise (page 79). Losing weight and getting more exercise will increase the proportion of HDL—which may be particularly important for women. Recent research indicates that they may be at increased risk of heart attack with an HDL level under 45.

MONITORING YOUR PRESSURE

People who check their blood pressure regularly control it better than people who don't. They avoid nasty surprises, and can also see just how well their blood-pressure control measures are working. In the early stages of your campaign to bring your pressure down, get your pressure checked every two or three weeks. Later on, once a month is usually enough.

- Arrange for pressure to be measured by a nurse at your doctor's office or perhaps at work.
- Don't use automatic or coin-operated machines unless you know that they are being kept well adjusted.

Should You Buy Your Own Equipment?

There are plenty of blood-pressure monitoring devices on the market, including some that are quite inexpensive. Unfortunately, many are not very reliable.

Electronic machines are easiest to use, and some are accurate, but it is hard to check on their accuracy. Old-fashioned types are generally more reliable, and can be checked in the doctor's office. These have a dial on which you can read the pressure. The best have the stethoscope built into the cuff, and a metal ring that holds the cuff in a circle to make it easy for you to put it on your arm and tighten it with one hand.

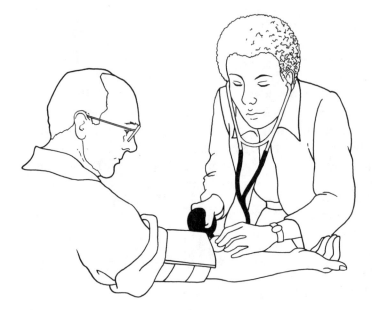

People who get their pressure checked regularly do a better job of keeping it under control.

If you plan to get your own equipment:

- Consult the doctor or nurse before you choose a model;
- Have the doctor or nurse show you how to use it.

Taking Your Blood Pressure

Remember that pressure goes up and down with activity, excitement, emotions, or for no particular reason.

- Take your pressure (or get it measured) at about the same time of day, when you have been sitting still for a while.
- Don't take it right after a walk, a cup of tea or coffee, or a meal. And don't take it when something exciting has just happened.
- Don't take it too often. You'll go crazy worrying about minor rises and falls. Remember, it's the average that counts.
- Ask the doctor whether and when you should report the numbers.

MEDICATION

Depending on the level of your pressure and what else is going on with your health, the doctor may or may not prescribe medication. In some cases, even if pressure is high, the doctor may want to work with you to try bringing the pressure down naturally first—then will prescribe medication only if natural measures don't work. In other cases, you may need medication right away. But even if you do, the doctor will also suggest that you take natural measures to reduce your pressure and help the medication do its job.

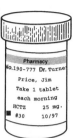

NOTE: Even if your high pressure is caused by some underlying disease, such as kidney disease, in all probability you will still have to work on lowering the pressure itself, just like everyone else with high pressure. There's unlikely to be a "magic bullet" that can "cure" your high blood pressure by removing the underlying cause.

Medication is not for everyone— but used right, it is a life- saver.

To Medicate or Not to Medicate?

The decision to use medication to treat high blood pressure should always be made carefully and thoughtfully. Whether or not your doctor prescribes medication will be based on your total medical situation. In general, the higher your average blood pressure is, the more you stand to benefit from medication. Most people with pressure above 160 systolic or 100 diastolic, or both, will need to be on medication. However, the level of blood pressure is not the only consideration. If you also smoke cigarettes or have a high cholesterol level, then the situation may be more urgent, and your doctor may use medication to bring your pressure down in a hurry (and will help you quit smoking and lower your cholesterol as well). Also, if the doctor finds evidence that your high pressure has begun to damage your heart or kidneys, it will be extra important to lower the pressure effectively and promptly.

You should always feel free to ask questions about your blood pressure treatment and the decision to prescribe (or not to prescribe) medication. After all, you are the one who will be taking the pills, so you should feel comfortable with the decision to use them. In some cases, you and your doctor may decide to wait a while, and see if losing weight, getting more exercise, and making dietary changes are enough to lower your pressure without help. Or you might decide to start a medication now, with the option to stop it in six months if you are successful in changing your lifestyle.

If you do take medication for your blood pressure, it is important to realize that this does not mean you are sick. The medication simply restores the normal setting to your blood-pressure control system. And fortunately there are a great many different medications that can do this.

What the Medications Do

Blood pressure medications save tens of thousands of lives every year, and they do it in different ways. There are three main types of medication:

1. **Diuretics,** which flush excess water and salt out of your system
2. **Beta blockers** and similar drugs, which act by altering the way the nervous system acts to control blood pressure
3. **Vasodilators,** which relax the blood vessels in different ways

The physician may start with one medicine, then move to another type if necessary. Sometimes you will have a combination of drugs. (To save money, ask your doctor or pharmacist if there are "generic" drugs that may be cheaper.)

How Drugs Interact

When prescribing blood pressure medication, the doctor will take into consideration any other drugs you are taking, such as birth control pills and insulin. **It is very important to tell the doctor about any medicine or drugs you take regularly, including street drugs.** Many blood pressure medications will not work in combination with other drugs, or the combination could be dangerous.

What about Side Effects?

Some blood pressure medications have no side effects or only minor ones. Others may have different side effects on different people. One person may have no major problems, whereas another might experience one or more of the following:

dizziness	headache
faintness	stuffy nose
skin rash	cramps
diarrhea	constipation
palpitations	impotence
breast tenderness	sleep disturbance

Ask the doctor what side effects you can expect. And if you *do* experience any, keep a record of when they happen and how severe they are. If they are really bad, call the doctor. Otherwise, wait until your next visit to discuss them. Don't suffer in silence! Your doctor can probably switch you to another drug that is just as effective and easier to live with. Or he or she may assure you that the side effects will soon pass. The bottom line is this: **Eventually, with the doctor's help, almost everyone can find a medication or combination of medications that will bring down blood pressure without significant side effects.**

Keeping Track

Here are some rules to follow, no matter what type of drug you are given:

- Make sure you know when you should take the medication and how (for example, before or after food).
- Make a note on your calendar to refill the prescription before it runs out.
- Make sure you have enough pills before you travel.
- Keep taking the medication **every day,** even if your pressure comes down and you feel fine.

Helping the Medication to Do Its Work

If you make the changes in lifestyle that your doctor suggests (which are probably the same as those you will find in this book), you will help the medicine to work and may even be able to cut down on the dosage eventually. In some cases, people can stop taking medication altogether. **But you should never stop taking medication without consulting with your doctor first.**

REMEMBER: There is no way that you can tell, just by the way you feel, whether your pressure is high or low.

Even if you have your own blood-pressure measuring device, and your pressure seems low and healthy, you can't tell what would happen if you stopped **taking** the medication.

Don't change your medication in any way. If you are wondering whether you still need the same dosage, always discuss it with your doctor. He or she may or may not say that it is safe to try a lower dosage.

The following checkup is for people who have been given blood pressure medication.

Checkup No. 2   YOUR MEDICATION

Has the doctor prescribed medication?   Yes ____   No ____

Name(s) of medication: 1. _____

2. _____

3. _____

Dosage (usually in mg):   1. _____

2. _____

3. _____

How many times a day: 1. _____

2. _____

3. _____

Special instructions (for example, with meals? before meals? bedtime?):

1. _____

2. _____

3. _____

Side effects expected
(ask the doctor):   Check if they happened

1. _____   _____

2. _____   _____

3. _____   _____

REMEMBERING YOUR MEDICATION

Here's a common scenario. In the beginning, you take your medication just the way the doctor prescribed it. But then you skip a pill or two. Then you go away for the weekend and forget to take your pills along. Or you run out, and it's several days before you have time to renew the prescription. Nothing much seems to happen. You don't feel sick, so you start forgetting your pills more often. And your pressure is soon back up, close to where it was before you began taking the medication.

Moral: Take your pills. Here are some tips to help you remember.

Pill-Taking Tips

Check the tips that you plan to use:

_____ Put the pills where they are linked to a part of your routine.
- Put them near your toothbrush or razor.
- Put them where you eat breakfast.

_____ Write reminders. Change the reminders every week; otherwise, you might get so used to them that you stop noticing them.
- Put a reminder on your bathroom mirror or the refrigerator door.
- Put a reminder on the door where you let the cat out (or in).

_____ Set your watch to beep at pill-taking time.

_____ Ask your nearest relatives to remind you to take your medication.

_____ Buy a "medication organizer" at your drugstore, with a compartment for each day. This is especially useful if you are taking more than one type of pill regularly.

_____ Set up a system for renewing the prescription.
- Make a note of the renewal date on your calendar.
- If your pharmacist will cooperate, give him or her a stack of reminder cards to mail to you.

_____ If you travel frequently, put reminders with your baggage.
- Fasten a note to your suitcase or travel kit to remind you to pack your pills.
- Travel with a spare prescription, in case you forget them.

To get pills into your body regularly, plan to get the thought of them into your head.

Remember: The pills are not magic. They need help from you if they are to work as efficiently as they can. So even if you are on medication (and certainly if you are not), plan to reduce your pressure naturally, following the advice in the rest of this book.

Part 2

What Changes Do You Need to Make?

Before you make changes in lifestyle, it's a good idea to know exactly what it is you most need to change. Then you can plan changes systematically. This part of the book includes a master checkup that will help you realize what changes you need to make, and what order you will make them in.

To help you with your answers, here are some reminders about the causes of high blood pressure and the factors that can make it more dangerous.

First, most people with high blood pressure have one or more of the following problems:

- They have close relatives with high blood pressure.
- They are sensitive to sodium and get too much of it (they may also get too little potassium, which is a helpful mineral).
- They are overweight.

23

In addition, they may make the situation worse in one or more of these ways:

- They may be generally out of shape and in need of exercise.
- They may be under stress.
- They may be boosting their pressure chemically with too much caffeine, alcohol, or other drugs.

Finally, some people with high blood pressure have other problems that need urgent attention, because of their risk of a heart attack. High blood pressure alone can double your risk of a heart attack or a stroke. High cholesterol may double it again, giving you four times the risk. And if you smoke, you may double the risk one more time, giving you a very high risk indeed. So a reduction in cholesterol—and quitting smoking—can be an important part of your treatment plan.

IDENTIFYING YOUR OWN RISK

The first step toward blood pressure control is to identify what's going on in your body, your life, or your family history that may be making (or keeping) your pressure high. The master checkup that follows will help you identify your own problems.

Checkup No. 3   MASTER CHECKUP

Add up the points, and see what might be affecting your blood pressure. First, there's one factor you can't do anything about:

Family *Give yourself one point if a parent, brother, or sister had (or has) high blood pressure.*	

Next, here are five factors you *can* control:

Weight *Pinch the flesh at the side of your waist (thumb on top of the fold).* *Give yourself one point for each inch you can pinch.*	
Salt *If you salt food at the table, give yourself one point.* *If you often eat salty snacks like chips, nuts, or pretzels, give yourself another point.* *If you use prepared foods like frozen dishes, soups, sauces, or mixes (and don't pick low-sodium types), or often eat out at fast-food restaurants, give yourself one more point.*	
Exercise *If you don't walk (or do other exercise) three or four days a week for at least 20 minutes on each of those days, that's one point. If you are a real couch potato, two points.*	
Stress *If you feel uncomfortably stressed more than once a day, give yourself a point.*	
Chemicals *A little coffee or alcohol probably won't affect your blood pressure, but if you think that you are revving up your motor with too much caffeine, alcohol, or other drugs, give yourself a point.*	
Total	

USING THE MASTER CHECKUP

The checkup can't tell you everything that could be affecting your blood pressure, but it can help you see where some of your own problems might lie. It will also give you a "baseline" against which you can measure the

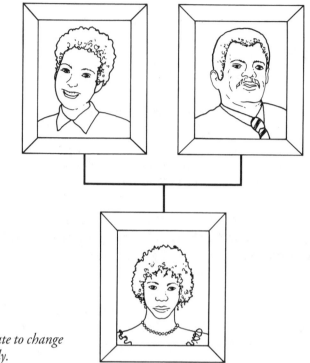

It's a bit late to change your family.

changes you make in your diet and lifestyle. After you have worked through this book, you will find another copy of the checkup (on page 125). Your goal is to reduce your point total by the time you get there. And look on the bright side. The more points you earned in the checkup, the more opportunities you will have to improve your score—and your health.

Where to Start?

If you have inherited the tendency to develop high blood pressure, changing your parents might be the most effective thing you can do. But it's a little late for that, so we will suggest that you start with the two other major areas of change:

- Reduction in sodium (and an increase in potassium, which is the helpful mineral)
- Reduction in weight

The section on reducing weight will give you additional benefits: It will show you how to cut down the amount of fat you eat, which in turn can help reduce the effects of high blood pressure on your arteries by lowering the level of cholesterol in your blood.

People who are not overweight may choose to start with the sodium and exercise sections. Exercise is helpful in blood pressure control whether you are overweight or not—and it can be powerfully effective in reducing stress, as you will find when you work through the stress-control section. Reducing stress can help some people reduce or control their pressure. It can also help make life more pleasant, and can free up energy for making the other changes recommended in this book.

In each of the different "change" sections starting on page 33, you will find:

- Explanations about why these changes can be important to your health;
- Self-assessments that help you see what *you* need to do;
- Practical step-by-step programs to help you make changes, one step at a time.

Pacing Yourself

As you will see, making changes isn't something you should do too quickly. Here are two contrasting ways of going about it:

1. Pete, a compulsive character, reads through the sodium section, throws all foods containing salt out of his house, changes his food-buying habits in a big hurry—and by Tuesday, feels almost salt-free. Wednesday, he starts on weight—throws all food containing fat out of the house, adjusts his food-buying habits yet again, and makes a big switch in the food he orders in restaurants.

   By Friday morning, he's ready for exercise—and spends much of the weekend taking brisk walks. By Monday he's gasping for air, and the sudden changes in food have left him feeling seriously deprived. He's more than ready for the stress section.

2. Barbara decides to tackle her problems more systematically. She works through the sodium section and the weight section together so that she can coordinate food buying and preparation, gradually reducing sodium and fat at the same time. As part of the weight-control program, she starts walking. After a few weeks, she works through the exercise section to help her make walking a comfortable part of her routine. She also checks the stress section and makes some adjustments to help her cope with stressful situations—but

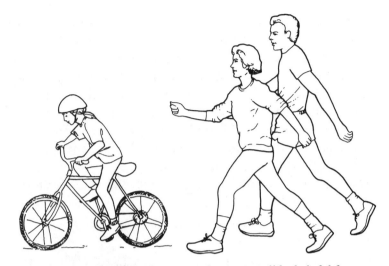

Get your family to make changes with you. It will be helpful for you, and they'll thank you—eventually.

realizes that she has already discovered one of the best natural tranquilizers in the world, in the form of walking.

Some people can "will" themselves into making rapid changes in their lifestyle. Sometimes this can work. But most people will be more successful in the long run if they approach the business of change as Barbara did, not taking on too much at a time.

Gradual change is more likely to last. For example, if you stop eating salt all at once, food will taste awful. But if you cut down gradually, you will be able to *unlearn* your taste for salt little by little, until you positively prefer the natural tastes of unsalted foods. And the same is true for other adjustments to food and lifestyle. You need time to unlearn old habits, and start to like new ones.

Don't Go It Alone

Changing your routine will be much easier if the rest of the family can make changes too. And even if they don't have high blood pressure, their health will improve because they are eating better and exercising more.

- Cutting down on salt will improve everyone's health—**especially the health of people who may have inherited your tendency to develop high blood pressure.**

- There are probably other members of your family who could use more exercise. Take them along; they'll all benefit.

- If you need to reduce your weight, you won't "go on a diet," so there is no need for you to eat food that's different from the type of food the rest of the family eats, except that you will probably find yourself eating less of the fat and more fruits, vegetables, and food from grains. That way of eating is recommended for everyone, whether they have high blood pressure or not, and whether they are overweight or not. If you can encourage the whole family to eat less fat (and more of the healthy stuff), you will be doing them all a favor.

WORKING ON YOUR ATTITUDE

There will be times in the first few months when you hit roadblocks. For various reasons, your enthusiasm for making changes may weaken. When that happens, you will need to be on your guard. An occasional treat, or some days off from exercise, is not going to hurt you. The trouble is that for some people a treat mysteriously becomes a daily event, or the day off from exercise accidentally stretches into a week or a month, and before they know it, they are back where they started.

Here is a thought that can help: Most people don't have to worry about sticking to their plans for more than six months or a year.

Why? It's not because their blood pressure problem disappears. Even if your numbers come down, there will always be a tendency for them to go up again, unless you keep up with the changed lifestyle (and the medication, if you need it). It's because after a while you will *like* what you are doing.

- Exercise won't seem like a chore; it will be something you enjoy.
- Salt won't seem an essential part of food. After you have cut down, you won't like it. Salty snacks and foods will taste bad.
- Cutting down on high-fat foods as you lose weight won't seem such a problem. You will learn to prefer foods that don't coat your mouth with grease.

In other words, stick with the advice in this book for the first few months. After that, your body should be on automatic pilot, doing what it likes— and staying healthy.

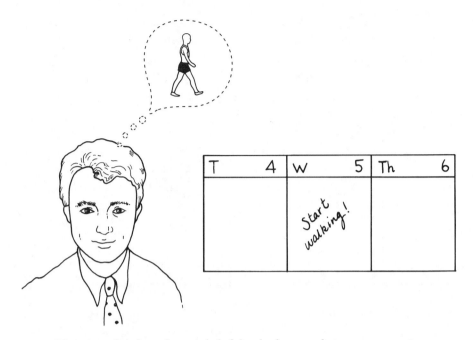

Planning ahead can be very helpful, whether you do it on paper or in your head.

To help with those first few months, here are some tips.

MAKING A PLAN

Some people keep plans in their head. Others like to plan on paper. If you like to write out your plans, you could get a large wall-calendar with a square for each day of the year, and plan out your major changes, week by week.

Don't Get Taken by Surprise

If an event is coming up that might make it hard to avoid high-fat, high-sodium foods, take some time to think of how you will cope. For example:

- If you will be eating in restaurants, carry a list of selections that won't overload you with sodium and/or fat (see pages 50 and 70 for eating-out information).

- If you might be heading into a high-temptation social situation, like a family reunion or holiday party, practice politely refusing food that your body doesn't need.

- If something comes up that might make it difficult to stick to your eating and exercise plans (like a business trip), spend some time looking for alternatives. Pack your walking shoes, or check on the availability of swimming pools, or plan hotel breakfasts that won't be too high in fat and sodium.

- If you *do* find that you are taken by surprise, and the circumstances trip you up, don't waste time feeling guilty. Just start off the next day as if there had been no break in your new routine.

Get Social Support

Show the following note to your spouse or whoever is most likely to be helping you with the changes in your diet and lifestyle.

A Note for Your Spouse or Other Helper

If someone close to you has high blood pressure, this is something to take seriously—but it's not the end of the world. Wonderful progress has been made in treating the condition.

Whether a person with high blood pressure is taking medication or not, the advice in this booklet will be important in helping get that blood pressure under control. *You* can help in the following ways:

- Read through this book so that you can make helpful suggestions for things to eat or for types of exercise you can do together.

- If the person with high blood pressure wants gentle reminders, make gentle reminders.

- Don't treat the person as if he or she is sick—think of it as *preventing* illness. Once the high blood pressure is under control, your spouse, friend, or relative may be stronger and healthier than ever.

- Don't nag. Instead, give positive feedback when you notice changes or improvements.

- Don't expect sudden changes. We advise the person who is working through this book to make changes in diet and lifestyle gradually, step by step, until the new and healthy way of living is second nature.
- Don't tell the person with high blood pressure what changes you think he or she should tackle next. But do be available to discuss plans.
- Don't make him or her feel different from the family, but do try to encourage others in the family to make the same changes. Everyone will be healthier if they follow the advice in this book.
- Be available any time the person with high blood pressure wants to talk, or complain, or hear helpful suggestions.

Part **3**

Change Sections

Here is a road map to the five "change sections" in this book:

Although we have put sodium first, remember that it is not the only factor that might require attention. We suggest you start on weight control and exercise before you complete the program for sodium reduction. And some people will also want to get started on stress, because high stress levels can make it hard to work on other changes.

Sodium

In some parts of the world, hypertension is almost unknown, and even elderly people have ideal blood pressure levels. Part of their good health may be due to the fact that they are usually lean, get a lot of exercise, and do not use alcohol. However, the most striking difference between them and us is that they have a very low intake of sodium, which we get mostly from salt.

Many people (including nearly all of those with high blood pressure) are highly sensitive to salt. It affects us like this:

- When we eat salt, the sodium in it goes mostly into our bloodstream, making it more salty.
- The body responds by adding more water to the blood, to return its level of saltiness to normal.
- The extra fluid increases the volume of blood, which in turn increases blood pressure.
- Eventually, the kidneys get rid of the excess sodium and water in the urine. But if salt-sensitive people continue to eat a high-salt diet, their blood pressure will stay high as a "cost" of getting rid of the extra sodium.

A large majority of people with high blood pressure can reduce pressure by going on a very low-sodium diet. Before modern drugs became available, such diets were the only way to treat hypertension. This is no longer the case, but most people with high blood pressure will be helped by reducing salt intake even if they are on medication. Indeed, worldwide studies of the relationship between blood pressure and sodium show that we would all be better off by eating less salt.

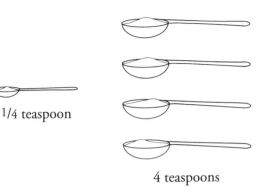

1/4 teaspoon

4 teaspoons

The average person gets about four teaspoons of salt each day but only needs a quarter teaspoon.

Our Need for Salt

Some people may be afraid that they will be going against nature if they stop eating salt, or cut down on the amount. After all, they say, don't wild animals trek hundreds of miles to the nearest salt lick? Doesn't that show that all animals, including us, need salt? True, we do need some sodium, which is in the salt. And if our diet consisted entirely of grass grown in a type of soil that doesn't put any sodium in it at all—as it does for those animals—you might see herds of humans thundering across the plains to get their salt fix. As it is, we get more than enough sodium in the foods we eat. **We don't need to add any.**

Your Goals for Reducing Sodium

Talk to your doctor about the amount of sodium you should aim for. Some people will need to keep their sodium intake very low indeed. Others will need only a moderate restriction. Here are some numbers, in milligrams:

Average daily intake of sodium	4000 mg
Average amount needed for good health	200 mg
Goal for moderate restriction	1800 mg
Goal for more thorough restriction	1200 mg
Average daily needed	200 mg

How does that translate into salt? To get to the level of 4000 milligrams of sodium, the average person eats the equivalent of four teaspoons of salt every day. **But all we really need each day is about 200 milligrams of sodium—which translates to less than a quarter teaspoon of salt!**

It's hard to get your intake of sodium that low, even if you don't add any salt at all, because you'll get more than 200 mg each day in foods that have sodium as a natural ingredient. So it's almost impossible for people to get less sodium than their bodies need, no matter how hard they try.

What about Sweat?

Do you have to add salt when you sweat a lot? It depends on what you mean by "a lot." Normal sweating can usually be taken care of with normal, low-sodium eating. If you sweat very heavily, then experts say it's okay to add a pinch of salt with your dinner—but you still don't need salt pills, salt supplements, or even as much salt as most people are eating normally in the course of a day. (The most important thing to do if you sweat heavily is to replace the water you have lost by having plenty to drink before, during, and after exercise, especially on a hot day.)

Un-Learning the Taste for Salt

Salt is an acquired taste. Babies eating their first salt are likely to express dislike. Even though salt is no longer added to commercial baby food (it was taken out, after an outcry by pediatricians and others), the child's parents often can't believe the baby likes food to taste so "bland" and they add salt. Before long, the baby is hooked.

If, like most babies, you went on to a childhood full of fast food and salty snacks—as well as plenty of salt in your meals at home—you have had many years to learn to like the taste. You may need a few weeks to un-learn it. So take your time.

How This Section Will Work

We'll start with a checkup to help you see how much salt you are eating now. After the self-assessment, you will find suggestions for reducing your sodium intake step by step. At each stage, some of the advice is appropriate for those who need to reduce sodium only moderately, and some will apply to those whose doctors suggest greater sodium restriction.

We will also suggest increases in potassium, which you can think of as the good mineral, helping to balance out the fluid levels in your body.

Keeping Track of Progress

Not everyone likes record keeping, but you may find it helpful to fill in the dates on this chart when you finish a step. Allow at least a week for each step that involves a change in the way you eat.

Step 1	Find out your sodium intake	_____ / _____ / _____
Step 2	Add less salt at the table	_____ / _____ / _____
Step 3	Cut down on salt in cooking	_____ / _____ / _____
Step 4	Shop for foods low in sodium	_____ / _____ / _____
Step 5	Eat more fruits and vegetables	_____ / _____ / _____
Step 6	Special circumstances	_____ / _____ / _____

STEP 1   FIND OUT YOUR SODIUM INTAKE

Your first step in sodium control will be to find out approximately how much sodium you are getting now.

Most of the sodium we eat comes in the form of added salt (sodium chloride). You may also be getting a significant amount of sodium in the form it appears naturally in foods (especially meat and cheese) and in other ingredients with "sodium" or "soda" in their names (like monosodium glutamate or baking soda).

Checkup No. 4 is a sodium self-test that will give you an idea of where most of *your* sodium is coming from. Complete the chart now, then work through the other steps in this section. At the end of the section, you will meet the same chart again—and by then, you will probably come up with some different answers.

Checkup No. 4   SODIUM SELF-TEST

ADDED SALT		
How many times a week do you add salt at the table?	___ more than 8 times	___ 3–7 times	___ 0–2 times
In cooking, do you use more or less salt than the recipe calls for?	___ more	___ about the same	___ less
Do you add MSG (Accent)?	___ more than once a week	___ about once a week	___ less than once a week
Do you use baking soda or baking powder?	___ more than once a week	___ about once a week	___ less than once a week
SALTED PREPARED FOODS		
How often do you use:			
Dry mixes (soup, hamburger extender, instant hot cereal, etc.)?	___ more than once a week	___ about once a week	___ less than once a week
*Bottled sauces (ketchup, mustard, soy sauce)?	___ more than once a week	___ about once a week	___ less than once a week
*Canned soups, gravies, or other prepared foods?	___ more than once a week	___ about once a week	___ less than once a week
Sausage, ham, or lunch meats (including turkey)?	___ more than once a week	___ about once a week	___ less than once a week
Salted snacks (nuts, chips, pretzels)?	___ more than once a week	___ about once a week	___ less than once a week
*Frozen dinners and side dishes?	___ more than once a week	___ about once a week	___ less than once a week

EATING OUT			
How often do you eat fast foods (pizza, burgers, chicken, fries)?	____ *more than once a week*	____ *about once a week*	____ *less than once a week*
*How often do you eat in **Asian restaurants?*	____ *more than once a month*	____ *about once a month*	____ *less than once a month*

Except low-sodium types.
***Except those that use no MSG or other high-sodium seasonings.*

Using This Chart

This chart can't give you a precise idea of the number of milligrams of sodium you get in a day, but it can suggest where you should make changes. The following steps will help you move your answers to the right.

STEP 2   ADD LESS SALT AT THE TABLE

In this step, you will start breaking the habit of adding salt at the table. People who have been in the habit of adding a lot of salt to food may spend more than a week on this step as they gradually get used to less salty food.

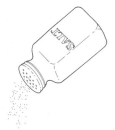

Remember that salt is an acquired taste—and for many of us, it has been covering up the true tastes of food for many years. As you cut back on the salt, you will rediscover those tastes.

Try shaking the habit, not the salt.

Check when you have completed these steps:

____ If you add salt to food before tasting it, STOP! Taste and think. Then add salt only if you really need it.

____ Once you are no longer salting food automatically, move the salt shaker off the table completely so that you have to get up and get it before adding any salt.

____ Stop adding salt to food completely.

NOTE: Some people may need to work through Step 3 (or ask whoever does the cooking to work through it) before they complete this one. You may need to add different seasonings to food before you can enjoy it with no salt.

When you have checked off the actions in this step (or if you didn't need to), move on to Step 3.

STEP 3   CUT DOWN ON SALT IN COOKING

This step is a bit more complicated than Step 2—partly because it might involve someone else, if you don't do your own cooking.
Sodium gets into food in the kitchen in three main ways:

- Through added salt
- Through high-sodium seasonings
- Through processed foods or ingredients (such as prepared sauces or mixes) that come from the manufacturer already stuffed with sodium

In this step, we deal with the first two problems: added salt and seasonings.

Added Salt

Recipes will call for a certain amount of added salt not because the dish will be a disaster without it but because we have all been trained to like the taste of salt. Now that you are untraining your taste buds in this respect, you can learn to prefer food with less salt. But don't rush it and cut out all salt at once. Take a few weeks to cut down the amount gradually.

Check when you have completed these steps:

____ Start by cutting the amount of salt in recipes in half.

____ After a few weeks, cut the amount in half again. For example, instead of a teaspoon of salt, add only a quarter teaspoon. (See the chart on pages 41–42 for seasonings you can use instead of salt.)

____ If the doctor has told you to go on a very low sodium diet, after a few weeks stop adding salt completely.

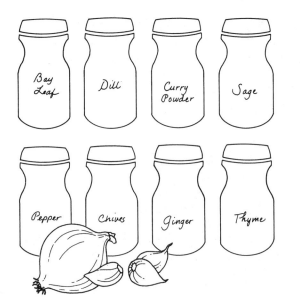

Food doesn't have to taste salty. Try exploring new seasonings.

Seasonings

As we have said before, when you are used to food without salt, you will like it. You will wonder why you ever interfered with the natural flavor of a fresh tomato, for example. But there will still be many foods or dishes that can use a little help—especially in the early stages, before you are fully ready for the most subtle of the natural tastes.

Use the flavor chart to explore new seasonings.

FLAVOR CHART
Alternatives to Salt

Meat	
Beef	Bay leaf, celery seed, dry mustard powder, green pepper, marjoram, fresh mushrooms, nutmeg, onion, oregano, pepper, sage, thyme
Lamb	Curry powder, garlic, mint, pineapple, rosemary
Pork	Apple, applesauce, garlic, onion, sage, savory, thyme
Poultry	
Chicken	Ginger, green pepper, lemon juice, marjoram, fresh mushrooms, paprika, parsley, sage, thyme

Fish	
Fish	Allspice, bay leaf, curry powder, dry mustard powder, lemon juice, marjoram, paprika, rosemary, tarragon

Vegetables	
Corn	Green pepper, pimiento, fresh tomato
Cucumbers	Chives, dill, garlic, vinegar
Green beans	Dill, lemon juice, marjoram, nutmeg, pimiento
Greens	Onion, pepper, vinegar
Peas	Green pepper, mint, fresh mushrooms, onion, parsley
Potatoes	Green pepper, mace, onion, paprika, parsley
Winter squash	Brown sugar, cinnamon, ginger, mace, nutmeg, onion
Tomatoes	Basil, marjoram, onion, oregano

Soup	
Bean soup	Dry mustard powder
Vegetable soup	Allspice, vinegar, dash of sugar
Pea soup	Bay leaf, parsley

Growing Herbs

Grow some herbs in the yard or on a windowsill. Hang up some to dry, and when they are crumbly, put them in jars. Or freeze them like this, to keep the taste fresher:

- Tie in a bundle
- Dip in boiling water for 10 seconds
- Plunge into ice water
- Dry, then remove leaves and freeze in sandwich bags

WARNING: All herbs and spices are fine for your health, including peppers in any strength. The following seasonings, however, are not fine— they are loaded with sodium:

Soy sauce (except for low-sodium)

Bouillon or bouillon cubes (except low sodium)

Ketchup and barbecue sauces

Monosodium glutamate, which appears under the brand name "Accent"

Most made-up seasoning mixes, such as poultry seasoning or Italian seasoning

Anything with "salt" in the name, such as garlic salt or celery salt

STEP 4   SHOP FOR FOODS LOW IN SODIUM

Many supermarket foods are loaded with salt. Luckily, new labeling laws make it easy to find where the sodium is hiding.

1. Nutrition labels on all processed food have to tell you how much sodium is in each portion.
2. Any food labeled "reduced sodium" or "low sodium" has to mean what it says. Specifically:

Reduced sodium	Must have 25% *less* sodium than found in the regular type of this food (which doesn't tell you much)
Low sodium	Less than 140 milligrams per serving
Very low sodium	Less than 35 milligrams per serving
Sodium free	No sodium—guaranteed

Making the Switch

To give your taste buds an adjustment period, don't move directly from a fully salted version of a food to one that is completely sodium free, but get there in stages. Try "reduced sodium" or "low sodium" before going all the way.

Checking Out the Supermarket

Give yourself extra time in a supermarket, and use it to read labels. Once you are in the habit of doing this, you will find it is easy to find products that are low in sodium or sodium free.

Check when you are regularly carrying out these steps:

_____ Read the **large** print on the labels.
   • Look for products labeled "reduced sodium," "low sodium," and "very low sodium."
   • Even if you are not ready to buy these yet, notice just how many of these foods are now available.

_____ Read the **small** print on the labels, and look for the amount of sodium. Here's a typical label of a can of chili with beans:

Nutrition Facts	
Serving Size 1 cup (265g)	
Servings per container about 2	
Amount per serving	
Calories 330	Fat Cal 140
	% Daily Value*
Total Fat 15g	23%
Sat Fat 6g	31%
Cholesterol 30mg	10%
Sodium 1050mg	44%
Total Carb. 30g	10%
Fiber 14g	54%
Sugars 7g	
Protein 18g	37%
Vitamin A 35%	Vitamin C 2%
Calcium 8%	Iron 20%
*Percent Daily Value (DV) is based on a 2000 calorie diet.	

It's easy to use food labels to compare the amount of sodium in different products so you can pick the brand with the least.

_____ Use the labels to compare quantities of sodium per serving in different brands.
   • If your regular brand of crackers gives you 400 milligrams or more of sodium per serving, look for a brand with a label that shows less.

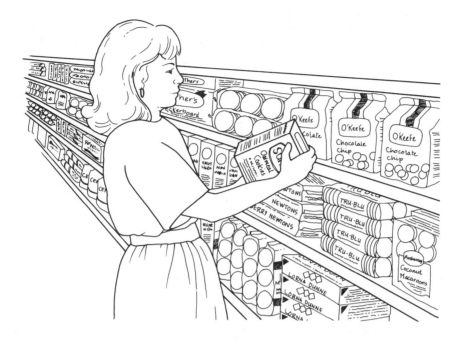

As you read your way through the grocery store, the labels will tell you all you need to know.

- Check the range of sodium quantities for a certain type of food—frozen dinners, for example. Their sodium may cover a very wide range, from well over 2000 milligrams all the way down to a few hundred.

____ Compare "percentage of daily value" for sodium that is given on product labels. Percentage figures may not be the best guides for people with high blood pressure, because they are calculated for people who *don't* have high blood pressure and can take up to 2400 milligrams of sodium in a day. But if percentage figures are very high, they can warn you to avoid those products.

____ To save yourself the trouble of reading labels, buy foods sold in their natural state, before any food company with a quick hand on the salt shaker has been able to get at them. As you will see from the shopping guidelines, coming up next, many prepared foods are very high in sodium.

SHOPPING GUIDELINES FOR SODIUM CONTROL

	Low Sodium	Medium Sodium	High Sodium
Breads	Most bread English muffins Bagels	Salted bread sticks Croutons Crumbs	
Cereals	Cooked cereals Some dry cereals (see labels)	Most dry cereals	Some bran cereals "Mix and eat" hot cereals
Crackers	Flatbreads Crispbreads Matzo	Graham crackers Oyster crackers Saltines	Pretzels Chips
Cheese	Farmers' cheese Ricotta Swiss cheese	Dutch cheese Mozzarella	Processed cheese Cottage cheese Roquefort, blue cheeses
Milk	Regular milk	Buttermilk	
Cakes, cookies, candies	Fig bars Ginger snaps Hard candy	Angel food cake Cake mixes	
Dessert	Frozen yogurt	Pudding mixes	
Fish	Fresh fish	Pre-breaded fish	Canned, dried, or smoked fish
Poultry	Fresh chicken or turkey		Processed poultry, such as turkey sausage
Red meat	Fresh meat		Corned beef; dried beef
Canned food			Canned soups; vegetables, stews
Packaged food			Frozen dinners Packaged foods like macaroni and cheese, meat extenders

	Low Sodium	**Medium Sodium**	**High Sodium**
Salad dressing	Homemade	Mayonnaise	French, thousand island, blue cheese, Italian; dry mixes
Soups	Homemade		Most canned and dry
Vegetables	Fresh	Frozen beans and peas	Canned vegetables Pickles Olives

NOTE: Check labels! Some foods in the high-sodium category may come in low-sodium versions.

STEP 5   EAT MORE FRUITS AND VEGETABLES

There are many excellent reasons for eating more fruits and vegetables, especially fresh. The two reasons that concern us here are these:

1. Fruits and vegetables are naturally low in sodium.
2. Fruits and vegetables (especially certain fruits) are naturally high in potassium.

The Low-Sodium Advantage

Remember that most sodium is added during processing. For example:

- The creator of the original tomato included only 4 milligrams of sodium.
- The person who canned the tomato added 160 milligrams per serving.
- When it got turned into sauce, it acquired a total of 530 milligrams per serving.
- When it was distilled down into ketchup, it received 126 milligrams—per tablespoon.

Here are some examples of the way sodium is added as food gets processed:

PROCESSED FOODS			FRESH FOODS		
	Amount	Sodium (milligrams)		Amount	Sodium (milligrams)
Tomato juice	1 cup	878	Fresh tomato	4 oz	4
Canned peas	1 cup	493	Fresh peas	1 cup	2
Potatoes au gratin	1 cup	485	Baked potato	1 cup	8

The lesson from all of this: When possible, buy fruit and vegetables unprocessed, and process them yourself (or eat them the way they come).

The High-Potassium Advantage

Fruits and vegetables have the advantage of giving you a good supply of potassium, which is helpful in regulating the fluid balance of the blood.

The Nutritional Advantage

Eating more fruits and vegetables every day will help control weight (see next section) and improve your general health.

The federal government, in its "Dietary Guidelines for Americans," recommends that everyone should eat at least two servings of fruit and three servings of vegetables a day. Here are some suggestions for ways to fit them into your life.

Check each tip when you have started following it (or if you follow it already):

—— Make a point of eating fruit at least twice a day, especially the types high in potassium (marked here with "*"):

apples*	melons*	pears
apricots	nectarines*	prunes
bananas*	oranges	strawberries
grapefruit	peaches	

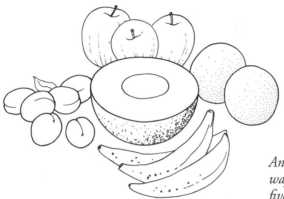

An apple a day gets you part-way there. Fruit and vegetables five times a day is better.

- Eat fruit as a snack.
- Have plain fruit for dessert.
- Drink fruit juice (*not* regular tomato juice, which is sky-high in sodium).

_____ Make a point of eating at least three servings of vegetables a day, preferably not overcooked (1 serving = ½ cup cooked or 1 cup raw). The following vegetables are especially low in sodium (and the potatoes are high in potassium):

broccoli	eggplant
brussels sprouts	potatoes
corn on the cob	squash

- Add a vegetable at lunch and dinner.
- Prepare celery, carrot, or zucchini sticks, and keep them in the refrigerator ready to eat as snacks.

Salads

Salads can be a nutritional booby trap. A green salad may provide barely more than a teaspoon of vegetable (once the lettuce is chewed up), but it can bring with it more than a tablespoon of high-sodium, high-fat salad dressing.

If you eat salads, put in a variety of vegetables besides lettuce, such as carrots, broccoli, and squash. Buy a low-fat, low-sodium dressing, or make your own, flavored with vinegar, lemon juice, yogurt, mustard, herbs, or garlic.

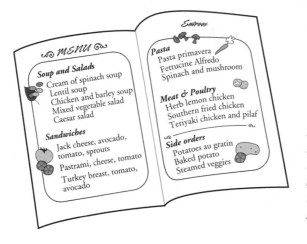

Rule 1 of eating out: Remember, you're paying the bill! Feel free to ask questions about items on the menu and to make special requests.

STEP 6 SPECIAL CIRCUMSTANCES

In this step, you will find out how to spot sodium when you are eating out or when sodium comes up under different names. These two problems may be related, because some forms of sodium in disguise (for example MSG— monosodium glutamate) may crop up most frequently in restaurants.

Eating Out

As you will see in the weight section (page 70), where the question of eating out is also addressed, you have one major trump card in restaurants: You (or someone you are with) will pay the bill. You have a right to find out what you are eating and to request food with less sodium.

1. Ask what's in the food. In some restaurants, this may mean asking whether certain ingredients are used, such as:

> Miso (in Japanese restaurants)
> Soy sauce (in Asian restaurants)
> Monosodium glutamate
> Meat tenderizer
> Heavy doses of garlic salt, onion salt, etc.
> High-sodium sauces

2. Be suspicious in fast-food restaurants.

   • As you can see, sodium adds up fast in the fast-food trade—even before someone salts your french fries.

Food	Quantity	Mg of Sodium
Cheese pizza	½ a 12-inch pizza	1347
Double cheeseburger	1	1000–1500
Roast beef sandwich	1	880

- If you eat often at fast-food places, ask for their printed nutrition information. Many of the chains are trying hard to cut down on sodium (though they still have a long way to go) and may have some choices that are within your range.

Hidden Sources of Sodium

In the effort to cut down on sodium, don't let yourself be sabotaged by one or two products that may be sky-high in the stuff, such as baking soda, baking powder, bicarbonate of soda, or even mineral water whose main mineral may be—guess what. (Read labels of soft drinks to see if significant amounts of sodium have crept in.)

FINAL SODIUM SELF-TEST   Checkup No. 5

Take this checkup and see how much you have changed since you first answered these questions (page 38).

ADDED SALT			
How many times a week do you add salt at the table?	___ more than 8 times	___ 3–7 times	___ 0–2 times
In cooking, do you use more or less salt than the recipe calls for?	___ more	___ about the same	___ less
Do you add MSG (Accent)?	___ more than once a week	___ about once a week	___ less than once a week

ADDED SALT		
Do you use baking soda or baking powder?	___ more than once a week	___ about once a week	___ less than once a week

SALTED PREPARED FOODS		
How often do you use:		
Dry mixes (soup, hamburger extender, instant hot cereal, etc.)?	___ more than once a week	___ about once a week	___ less than once a week
*Bottled sauces (ketchup, mustard, soy sauce)?	___ more than once a week	___ about once a week	___ less than once a week
*Canned soups, gravies, or other prepared foods?	___ more than once a week	___ about once a week	___ less than once a week
Sausage, ham, or lunch meats (including turkey)?	___ more than once a week	___ about once a week	___ less than once a week
Salted snacks (nuts, chips, pretzels)?	___ more than once a week	___ about once a week	___ less than once a week
*Frozen dinners and side dishes?	___ more than once a week	___ about once a week	___ less than once a week

EATING OUT		
How often do you eat fast foods (pizza, burgers, chicken, fries)?	___ more than once a week	___ about once a week	___ less than once a week
How often do you eat in **Asian restaurants?	___ more than once a month	___ about once a month	___ less than once a month

*Except low-sodium types.
**Except those that use no MSG or other high-sodium seasonings.

Weight

How does excess weight affect blood pressure?

It's a very complex relationship that we don't yet fully understand. For one thing, not everyone who is overweight has high blood pressure. Some people who are quite obese may have normal pressure, and some of those with high blood pressure may be positively lean.

But the bottom line is this: One of the most important causes of blood pressure is excess weight. So everyone with high blood pressure who is also overweight should consider losing some pounds.

The relationship between weight and high blood pressure starts early in life, and as many as half of all obese school children may already have high blood pressure.

Losing weight is not easy, as you may know if you have tried it before. But the effort will pay off. In many cases, blood pressure comes down by one point on the systolic scale for each pound lost.

If you are not yet on medication, controlling weight can help keep pressure down without it. If you *are* on medication, controlling or reducing weight can help the medication to work, or allow you and your doctor to consider reducing the dosage or stopping the medication altogether.

WHAT KIND OF WEIGHT?

When we talk about the advantages of losing weight, we don't always mean weight at all. In most cases, what you need to lose is **body fat.** Think of a linebacker on a professional football team. This man may be much heavier than what the charts recommend for someone of his height—but he might not be overweight at all, if he's mostly made of muscle.

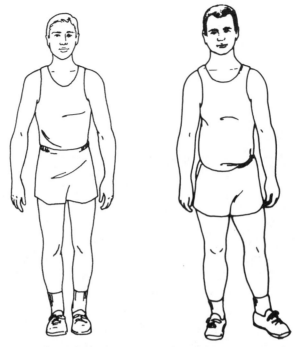

What you weigh can be less important than what you're made of.

In this section, we will help you to look leaner, fit into a smaller clothes size, and lose excess flab. You probably will lose weight as well.

First, take the checkup to help you see what *you* need to lose.

Checkup No. 6   WHAT HAVE YOU GOT TO LOSE?

Here are some questions to help you see if you have excess flab. Check which ones apply to you.

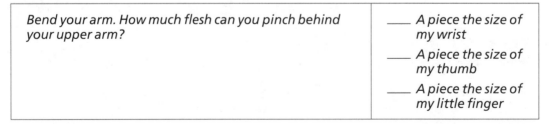

Bend your arm. How much flesh can you pinch behind your upper arm?	____ *A piece the size of my wrist*
	____ *A piece the size of my thumb*
	____ *A piece the size of my little finger*

How much flesh can you pinch on your side, at the waistline, with your thumb on the top of the fold?	____ 2 inches or more ____ 1 to 2 inches ____ Less than 1 inch
Look at yourself in the mirror, and be honest. Are those bulges flab or muscle?	____ Pure flab ____ Half and half ____ Muscle
How much more do you weigh now than you did at age 20? (Skip this question if you were overweight then or if you are a serious body-builder who has added heavy muscles.)	____ 20 pounds or more ____ 10 to 20 pounds ____ Less than 10 pounds
Look at a belt you have worn for several years. Did you have to move the buckle to a hole that made it longer? Or shorter?	____ I had to make it longer by more than one hole. ____ I made it longer by one hole. ____ It's the same as it was, or smaller.
Would your spouse (or equivalent) like you to lose weight?	____ Definitely ____ Probably ____ Not really

SETTING GOALS

If you need to lose weight, you'd probably like to take off eight to ten pounds in the first month, just like those smiling people in the commercials. This isn't likely to happen—or if it does, the weight is not likely to stay off (see later in this section). It is much better to lose weight slowly.

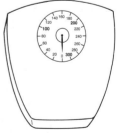

- Plan to lose about an inch of surplus flab at the waist within six to eight months.
- If you prefer to go by weight, aim to lose no more than one to three pounds a month.

Does that seem slow? Read on.

If you want to lose weight permanently, don't expect these numbers to change too fast.

How Not *to Lose Weight*

The worst way to lose weight is to go on a strict diet. You may follow the rules, suffer, and lose the weight, but chances are your strict diet has removed more than just the flab you wanted to get rid of. It has probably cut into your stock of good lean muscle tissue. And when you go back to normal eating (which has to happen, because no one can stick to a strict diet for long) weight may come back faster than ever. Why?

Because the muscle tissue you lost burned up more calories than flab, even when you were resting. So when less of you is made up of muscle, you need fewer calories to keep going.

And that's one reason why more than 90% of the time, diets fail completely, whether they are high-priced brand-name weight-loss programs, or diets from the latest "weight-loss miracle" book, or diets that your sister-in-law recommends, or just a cut in calories across the board. You go up and down in weight, year by year, struggling against yourself. And there is some evidence that this "yo-yo dieting" may be more harmful than just staying at your old weight.

How to Lose Weight

In this section, we offer a weight-control program that can get you to a *sensible* weight permanently. There are three basic rules.

Rule 1   Don't aim impossibly high. Some people who were slender as young adults may be able to get back to the shape they had at 20. Most can't. They will usually do better to settle for a moderate loss of weight—not a drastic one.

Rule 2   Don't try to lose weight by diet alone. A weight-loss program should *always* include some extra physical activity, if it is to work permanently.

Rule 3   Eat all the normal foods in moderate amounts, but try to cut down on **fat** whenever possible. That's the most concentrated source of calories. There is some evidence that the calories from fat really do turn into flab more easily than the calories from other foods. And your body doesn't need any added fat. There's more than enough for your needs already present in the grains, meats, and other foods you eat.

Rule 4 Eat at least three meals a day and at least two snacks. No need to go hungry.

How This Section Will Work

This weight-loss section has six steps:

1. Getting active
2. Cutting out the fat
3. Eating simple foods
4. Eating out
5. Trouble-shooting
6. Keeping the weight off

STEP 1 GETTING ACTIVE

How important is exercise? Many experts feel that it is almost impossible to lose weight permanently without it. When you cut down the supply of food, your body reacts as if it is threatened with famine. It slows down its metabolism to conserve the supply of fat and to help you get through this lean time. So even if you have put yourself on a very low-calorie diet, weight loss stops or slows to a crawl. That's why people may find it almost impossible to keep on losing through diet alone—and to keep the weight off—unless they cut their food to starvation levels, which is not healthy.

Exercise will help you to get over this "plateau" by burning up calories and by helping you hold on to your muscle tissue. Complete the following checkup to find out how much exercise you are getting now.

MINUTES OF ACTIVITY   Checkup No. 7

For this checkup, count only types of exercise that move your whole body along (standing for hours doesn't count for weight control, even if you are tired out at the end of the day). Come back to this checkup three months from now to see how many minutes of activity you have added.

1. How many minutes of exercise do you get as part of your normal routine (including work around the home)?

Activity	Minutes a Week	
	Now	In Three Months
Walking on the way to work		
Walking as part of work		
Digging		
Sweeping, vacuuming		
Mowing		
Other: _____		
Weekly total		

2. How much exercise do you get working out in a gym or at home?

Activity	Minutes a Week	
	Now	In Three Months
Aerobics, jazzercise, dance		
Treadmill		
Stair-stepper/exercise bike		
Rowing machine		
Cross-country skiing machine		
*Weights		
Other: _____		
Weekly total		

*Certain types of weight lifting can be harmful for people with high blood pressure. Talk to your doctor and a qualified trainer to develop a program that's safe and effective for you— or avoid muscle-building activities, and stick to programs that tone up your whole body.

3. How much exercise do you get in your leisure time outdoors?

Activity	Minutes a Week	
	Now	In Three Months
Walking (with or without dog)		
Jogging or running		
Bicycling		
Roller-blading		
Rowing		
Brisk swimming		
Other: _____		
Weekly total		

Now add up your weekly totals in all three categories: _____ _____

Remember to come back to this page three months from now to see how much your weekly activity has changed.

How to Add More Exercise

For most people, the simplest way to add more exercise is to do more walking. Walking is excellent for heart health, which may be important to you. Remember, people with high blood pressure have an increased risk of heart disease, and should try to reduce that risk whenever they have the opportunity.

Walking is also safe. Almost everyone can do it.

(If you want to start a form of exercise that's more demanding than walking, read the exercise section starting on page 79. There you will find some important safeguards and ways to select the most appropriate activity.)

Doing More Walking

Here are some suggestions for adding minutes of walking:

Check off any of these suggestions if they will work for you:

_____ Change your commute so that you walk for more of it. For example:
- Look into public transit; walking to and from the train or bus can help.
- Park your car so that you have to walk 10 minutes to where you are going.
- Think of something else that would work for you: _____
_____

_____ On breaks, take walks of 5 to 10 minutes.

_____ On the job, do any extra walking you can get away with.
- Walk to a co-worker's office instead of telephoning.
- Take the stairs instead of the elevator.
- When you have to run errands, go the long way round.
- Think of something else that would work for you: _____
_____

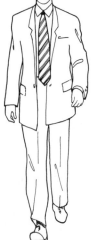

_____ At lunchtime, walk an extra 10 to 15 minutes.
- Walk to a restaurant.
- Walk to a park to eat your lunch.
- Eat at your desk, then walk (maybe with a co-worker).
- Think of something else that would work for you: _____
_____

A minute here, a minute there— pretty soon it adds up to a useful amount of walking.

_____ When you are shopping, train yourself not to move the car to go a couple of blocks. Leave it, and walk instead.

_____ Take 15- to 20-minute walks (or longer) to help you wind down after your day—perhaps with your family. Walking before meals can actually help take the edge off your appetite.

Keeping Track

For a few days, keep track of extra walking. Count anything that's more than about five minutes. Here's a sample:

Tuesday

Got off bus at Maple	10 min
Walked at break	5 min
Walked to lunch	10 min
Total	25 min

As you will see, a little here, a little there, and soon you are walking for a long distance every day. If you can manage an additional hour of walking or other exercise each day, so much the better. For ideas, look again at the checkup on pages 58–59 and see where you can fit in some more activity, by either walking or doing something you find more entertaining. Bicycling is great exercise for weight loss. Swimming is good exercise, but it's unlikely to take much weight off unless you do a great deal of it and keep up a good pace.

SAFETY NOTE: **If you do start anything more vigorous than walking or moderate bicycling, read through the information about safety on page 95 of the exercise section before you begin.**

Don't Stop There!

For some people, adding more exercise may be enough to solve the entire weight problem. Others will need help from diet—but getting more activity will make the diet part much, much easier.

STEP 2   CUTTING OUT THE FAT

In this step, you will pay special attention to one ingredient in food: fat. Even if you don't have much weight to lose, it makes sense to cut down on calories from fat. Remember, your high blood pressure has given you a higher-than-average risk of heart attack, and fat in the diet is one of the

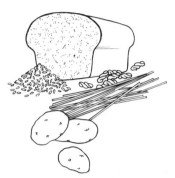

The good news—these foods rich in complex carbohydrates can fill you up without a lot of calories.

main causes of heart disease. Also, there is some early evidence that a high-fat diet may contribute directly to driving up blood pressure.

The most harmful fat, from your heart's point of view, is saturated fat. That's the type that comes from meat and dairy products, from tropical oils, and from other oils that have been "hardened" or "hydrogenated," like the vegetable oils in shortening or margarine. However, it is wise to limit *all* fat, both for weight control and for general health.

In case you are wondering about what's left to eat, there is good news. The starchy foods, like bread, potatoes, noodles or rice, are not fattening, in *moderate* quantities. Bite for bite, these foods are relatively low in calories (unless you add fat) and have the advantage of filling you up, as well as being good for your general health.

Fat Control

Read through the suggestions on the fat-control tips that follow and check off those you plan to use.

Meat, Fish, and Poultry

____ Cut down on the number of times you eat red meat (even the lean part contains hidden fat).
  • Aim to eat beef, lamb, or pork only three or four times a week to begin with, then cut down to once or twice a week.
  • Replace some meat dishes with chicken or fish, or with starchy main dishes made from beans, lentils, grains, and pasta.

_____ When you do eat meat, reduce the serving size.
- Think of meat as a flavoring rather than as a main course (for example, with spaghetti, beans, or rice, or in a vegetable stir-fry).
- Limit servings to the size of a deck of cards (three to four ounces).

_____ Eat lean cuts, such as pork tenderloin or flank steak.
- Trim as much fat as possible.
- Cook in a way that lets you discard the fat (i.e., broil, barbecue, or roast on a rack).

_____ Avoid hamburger if possible. If you do have it, buy extra-lean (or ask for a lean cut to be ground for you).

_____ Instead of high-fat prepared meats like sausage and luncheon meats, choose lower-fat types, like turkey. (You may be tempted by low-fat versions of high-fat prepared meats, such as turkey sausage, turkey ham, and so on. Beware! The processors tend to make up for the lack of fat by loading these products with sodium.)

_____ Take the skin off chicken or turkey before you eat it.

_____ Don't fry chicken or fish.

Dairy Fat

_____ Switch from whole milk or low-fat (2%) milk to 1% milk or nonfat. (Low-fat milk sounds healthy, but less than half the fat has been removed.)
- One percent and nonfat milk have just as much calcium as regular milk. They are fine for all members of the family over age 2.
- Don't make a big change all at once (i.e., whole milk to nonfat). You won't like it. Instead, step down gradually. Spend one or two weeks drinking 2%; then 1%; then, if you like, nonfat. (If you drink a glass or more of milk a day, go with the nonfat.)

_____ Eat yogurt, preferably nonfat. If you want low-fat frozen yogurt, check the labels (see "Reading Labels" on page 65). Some types are much higher in fat than others.

_____ Use plain nonfat yogurt instead of sour cream.

_____ Cut down on regular cheeses, which are high in fat as well as sodium. Look for low-fat, low-sodium types of cheese, reading labels carefully. Low-fat cheese should have three grams of fat or less per ounce.

Baked Goods

_____ If baked goods have labels, read them. Look for fat-free or low-fat baked goods (two grams or less of fat per serving).

_____ Most of the time, stick to bread-type foods such as fresh-baked breads, English muffins, bagels, breadsticks, and so on (*not* regular muffins—they often have as much fat as donuts).

Snack Foods

_____ Eat pretzels, fat-free chips (in unsalted versions), or air-popped popcorn without butter instead of regular chips and nuts. Even better, snack on vegetables.

_____ If you want candy, pick types that are made of sugar, like hard candy, instead of fat and sugar, like chocolate bars.

_____ Avoid regular ice cream. Instead, choose sherbet (sorbet), juice bars, or nonfat frozen yogurt.

Fats and Oils

_____ In cooking, cut the amount of fat and oil you use by at least half.

_____ Use nonstick pans. If they need a little oil, squirt them with a spray product or rub with oil.

_____ Don't fry—especially if the food is breaded.

_____ Cut the amount of butter or margarine on bread or toast in half (or find a substitute).

_____ Use low-fat or fat-free salad dressings.

Frozen Dishes

_____ Read the labels of frozen dishes or complete dinners. There are now plenty of low-fat choices.

Reading Labels

As you saw in the sodium section, the "nutrition facts" on food labels give very complete information. Almost all processed foods now tell you *exactly* how much fat is in the product. The information includes:

The size of a serving;
The number of grams of fat per serving;
What proportion of an average person's daily "value" for fat is provided
    by one serving.

NUTRITION FACTS		
Serving Size: 1 entree		
Servings per container: 1		
Amount per serving		
Calories 280	Fat Cal 70	
		% Daily Value*
Total Fat 8g		**12%**
Sat Fat 5g		**25%**
Cholesterol 70mg		**23%**
Sodium 800mg		**33%**
Total Carb. 38g		**13%**
Fiber 3g		**12%**
Sugars 2g		
Protein 14g		**37%**
Vitamin A 6%	Vitamin C 6%	
Calcium 10%	Iron 15%	
*Percent Daily Value (DV) is based on a 2000 calorie diet.		

Aunt Em's
Linguine
with
Clams

There's no need to guess whether a product is low in fat. You can read all about it.

The figure giving the percentage of the daily fat "value" may be misleading, because it implies that fat is good for you. It's true that your body needs some, but you don't need to add any from fats and oils or from prepared foods—there's enought fat for your needs hidden away in basic foods like grains.

The information on grams of fat, on the other hand, is very useful. Even if you wouldn't recognize a gram if you met it on the street (it's actually about 1/28th of an ounce), you can compare the number of grams between one brand and another. Or you can set "gram goals" for yourself. Many nutritionists suggest that you avoid anything that lists more than three grams per serving—except for complete frozen entrees, which can run up to 10 grams per serving. (If you can find food with one gram or less per serving, so much the better.)

Fighting Heart Disease

From the point of view of weight loss, fat is fat. It all has nine calories per gram (compared to four per gram for starches and protein). From the point of view of your heart, however, the most harmful fat is "saturated" fat. This is mostly fat from animals but includes some other types too.

There are high levels of saturated fat in:

The fat of beef, lamb, and pork;
Fat from cream, included in milk, butter, yogurt, cream, and cheese;
Tropical oils, such as coconut oil and palm oil;
Oils that have been hardened or hydrogenated during processing.

When you do add any fat, it's smart to avoid those sources of saturated fat. Stick to liquid oils (like corn, olive, or peanut oil). And the fat from fish and poultry is not as bad as the fat in red meat—it is much less saturated.

BUT from the point of view of weight loss, it makes sense to cut down on fat or oil in *any* form. It's all very high-calorie stuff.

STEP 3   EATING SIMPLE FOODS

For weight control, for sodium control, and for general heart health, the best foods are the ones that grow from the soil and that have not been overprocessed since they were harvested. These foods are not only low in fat but also high in bulk so that they make you feel full. They help your digestion keep working smoothly and also provide plenty of protein, vitamins, and other nutrients.

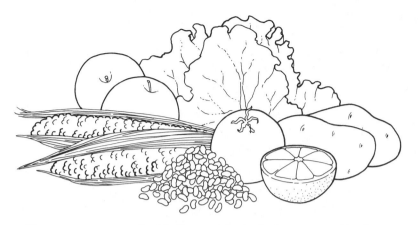

If you can get to your food before somebody else has processed it, there will be no surprise ingredients to trip you up.

In this section, we urge that you eat more food from grains:

> Bread
> Pasta
> Rice
> Grains like couscous, oatmeal, kasha

And food from vegetables:

> Green vegetables, especially leafy ones like spinach
> Root vegetables, including potatoes
> Red and yellow vegetables, including corn
> Dried vegetables like beans and lentils

And food from fruit:

> Berries and grapes
> Orchard fruits
> Tropical fruits, including bananas
> Melons, such as cantaloupe and honeydew

If you have already worked through Step 5 of the sodium section, you may have added fruits and vegetables to your daily diet to help with your potassium level. Look at page 47 of that section for ideas for eating more fruit and vegetables. Here, we will give you ideas for eating more food from grains. Remember, moderate amounts of bread, rice, potatoes, and pasta are not fattening, unless you add fat. And by taking the place of high-fat foods, they can help keep calories under control.

Serving Size

Once you have lost weight, and are eating to keep it off (with the help of exercise), you probably will not have to worry about serving size. Until then, here is a guide:

Vegetables	As much as you like
Fruit	As much as you like
Bread	Two slices at a meal, one as a snack
Rice	One cup of cooked rice (take more if you are really hungry)
Pasta	One cup, cooked

Adding More Food from Grains

In addition to five servings of fruits and vegetables, the U.S. government's nutrition guidelines call for us to eat between 6 and 11 servings of food from grains every day. Here are some ways you can fit in those grain servings.

Check those tips that look good to you.

_____ Have a fat-free low-sodium cereal for breakfast (like oatmeal).

_____ Add toast, English muffins, or toasted bagels (with jelly instead of butter).

_____ Carry a bread-type snack (such as salt-free pretzels or breadsticks).

_____ At lunch, aim for at least one serving of a grain food (for example, the bread part of your sandwich).

_____ At dinner, aim for at least two servings of grain foods (for example, bread and rice, or bread and pasta).

_____ For evening snacks, eat fat-free unsalted corn or wheat chips, or air-popped popcorn without added salt or butter.

Adding Fiber

You may have heard claims that added fiber can reduce your weight. These are probably not true—but food that is high in fiber can certainly help make the process of cutting calories more pleasant, because the fiber helps you to feel full (as well as keeping your digestion in good working order). One type of fiber (called "soluble"), which comes in oatmeal, apples, and other foods, can also help reduce levels of cholesterol.

Check those tips that look good to you.

____ When you buy bread, check the list of ingredients. Look for loaves that list a whole grain as the first item in the list (whether it is whole wheat or whole something else).

____ Try brown rice. It takes a little longer to prepare, but it's higher in fiber and also tastes good.

____ Leave vegetables and fruits as intact as possible. Don't skin them unless you have to.

____ Don't overcook vegetables. It's best to eat them raw or lightly cooked (steamed is best—boiling leaches the nutrients into the water).

"Meatless" Meals

Here's a quick way to cut down on the fat in your life and to lose weight: Increase the number of meals with *no* red meat, chicken, fish, eggs, or cheese. In other words, eat some meals each week that are vegetarian in the strictest sense.

Start with breakfast, which will give you seven weekly meals that are meatless, eggless, and cheeseless. Add two or three lunches or dinners that are based entirely on food from plants. Then maybe more.

Some people may be afraid to skip the protein that comes from meat, eggs, and dairy products. There's no need to worry. Even people who eat no food at all from animal sources can get all the nourishment they need if they eat a wide variety of vegetable foods, including whole grains and legumes such as beans, lentils, and peas. In fact, they may have a better chance than meat-eaters of living long, healthy lives. And they have less trouble controlling their weight.

Here are some ideas for meatless main meals:

Bean salads
Bean soup
Lentil soup

Pilafs made with lentils and bulgur
Vegetarian chili
Spaghetti with marinara sauce
Vegetable stew with potatoes
Curried vegetables on rice
Veggie-burgers (sometimes called "garden burgers")
Stir-fried vegetables on rice or noodles

(See the Suggestions for Further Reading on page 131 for books with vegetarian recipes.)

What about Sugar?

Sugar is not particularly fattening. Its main problem is that it is not particularly useful. It doesn't make you feel full; it doesn't provide any useful nutrients; in other words, it gives you calories you don't need and nothing else. But if you crave a sweet treat, go ahead—as long as the sugar doesn't come packaged with a lot of fat, as it does in candy bars, regular ice cream, and most cookies, pie, and cake.

Here are some good low-fat sweet foods. Check labels to find others that are low in fat.

Nonfat frozen yogurt	Sherbet
Jello	Fig bars
Juice bars	Angel food cake
Fudgesicles™	Ginger snaps
Hard candies	Meringues
Marshmallows	Fat-free cookies
Canned fruit	Fat-free cake

STEP 4 EATING OUT

For people who have to eat out much of the time, weight control (and fat control and sodium control) can present a major problem.

It's fine to have a great restaurant meal on a special occasion. The trouble is that for many Americans, eating in a restaurant is no longer a special occasion. In fact, many of us eat a third of our meals away from home! So for every day (or every week) restaurant eating, it's smart to plan meals that won't fill you with fat and sodium.

Suggestions for cutting down on **sodium** in restaurant food are on page 50. In this section, we will concentrate on **fat.**

Getting Started

There are guides available that list the calories or fat content of fast foods and other restaurant food. Here you will find a few suggestions to get you started on cutting down on fat when you eat out.

- On special occasions, when you want to spoil yourself, go for one high-fat food—and maybe split it with someone. Then balance it with selections that are low in fat. (And plan to use up some of those extra calories in exercise.)

- If you eat out very often, the high-fat food is not such a good idea, but you will soon develop a list of alternatives that are just as tasty, and that don't give you a lot of fat.

Fast-Food Restaurants

Fast-food places usually have low-fat choices available.

- Ask for printed nutrition information, and take it home to read.

- Choose foods that aren't fried in batter or smothered in cheese (a plain hamburger is a better choice than the deep-fried chicken or fish).

- Be cautious as you approach healthy-sounding offerings like baked potatoes. If potatoes are loaded with cheese and/or sour cream or a meat-based sauce, scoop out some of the stuffing.

- Choose salads that let you add the dressing yourself. Use a low-calorie (low-sodium) dressing if one is available—or take very little dressing, keep it on the side, and dip your fork in it to get some of the flavor.

- In pizza restaurants, order a thick-crust pizza with half the cheese (but watch out for heavy doses of sodium). Choose vegetable toppings rather than sausage.

- Look for low-fat versions of high-fat items (for example, turkey hot dogs instead of regular. But watch out for sodium!)

"Regular" Restaurants

Remember, *you* are paying the bill. If the restaurant wants to keep your business, it should make an effort to reduce the amount of fat on your plate, if you ask.

Here are some tips for eating out.

- While you are waiting, eat bread (but not butter).
- Order a la carte—not whole dinners.
- Pick a simple appetizer, such as a fruit cocktail, slice of melon, or green salad (with dressing on the side).
- If you want soup, avoid cream types. (And watch out for sodium in broth-based soups.)
- For the main course, choose fish or poultry that has been broiled, roasted, poached, or steamed:
  - Avoid dishes described as creamed, crispy, breaded, deep fried, pan fried, or sautéed.
  - Be suspicious of made-up dishes such as stews or casseroles that may have mystery ingredients.
- Ask for sauce or gravy to be served on the side so that you can take as little or as much as you like.
- If you choose spaghetti or noodles with a high-fat meat or cheese sauce, ask if you can have the sauce on the side. And ask for plenty of pasta (otherwise, you may find your dish is mostly sauce).
- Consider a vegetarian entree, if it isn't heavy on cheese or other high-fat dairy products.
- Feel free to ask for your vegetables to be prepared without cream, butter, or other sauces.
- Have fruit for dessert. Or if you crave something special, order one rich dessert and share it.

Here's a summary:

Good Words on the Menu	Not So Good
Broiled	Fried
Boiled	Sautéed
Poached	Crispy
Barbecued	Creamed
Steamed	Breaded
Baked	Grilled with fat

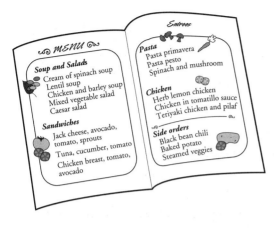

It helps to know which words on the menu are good news—and which words mean that a dish is full of fat.

Ethnic Restaurants

Here are some tips to help you order low-fat food in ethnic restaurants:

Chinese   Instead of fried rice, and other fried items, go for steamed rice, wonton soup, vegetable or chicken stir-fry—and perhaps one high-fat dish to share. *(Sodium reminder: Ask for food without MSG, and easy on the soy sauce.)*

Italian   Pasta is excellent for your health, especially the way Italians eat it —more pasta than sauce.

- Instead of fried dishes, or dishes made with a lot of cheese, go for pasta with tomato, marinara, or clam sauce.
- Try other marinara dishes (like shrimp).
- Don't add Parmesan cheese. It adds to the sodium as well as the fat.

Mexican   There are good Mexican choices that don't overload the food with lard, cheese, or sour cream. For example:

>Chicken, beef, or vegetable fajitas
>Black bean soup
>Gazpacho
>Chicken tacos
>Salsa, tortillas, Mexican rice
>Black beans (instead of refried beans)

Deli   If you pick up your lunch at a deli, your main hazards may be in the processed meats such as luncheon meats and sausage. These are very high in fat and sodium.

- Choose sandwiches made with unprocessed turkey or chicken, lean roast beef, or roast pork. *(Sodium reminder: Watch out for ham, tuna, pastrami, and processed turkey—they're low in fat, but high in sodium.)*
- Instead of mayonnaise in your sandwich, moisten it with a slice of tomato.
- Don't have cheese and meat on the same sandwich.
- If your deli piles on the meat, ask for half the amount and make up for it with extra lettuce, sprouts, or tomato.

STEP 5   TROUBLESHOOTING

People who don't need to lose weight often make it sound easy. "All you have to do is eat less." "All you have to do is exercise more." Simple, right? Right.

In real life, you are bound to run into roadblocks. Food is something we have to face at least three times a day, and eating (or not eating) can have a powerful effect on our mood and our willpower, as well as on our fat cells. (That's yet another reason for exercise—it can have an excellent effect on mood. See the next section.)

Here are some suggestions for keeping your body reasonably happy while you lose weight:

- Always eat three main meals. Don't skip breakfast (or lunch or dinner).
- At each meal, include some substantial food like bread, cereal, potatoes, rice, or noodles. (Don't take the "diet plate" consisting of a lettuce leaf and blob of cottage cheese! You'll be hungry again within a short time.)
- Choose whole-grain breads, which will keep you satisfied longer than baked goods made with overrefined flour.
- Don't fill yourself up completely at meals, because there's a gap between the time you finish eating and the time you feel completely full. Get up from the table and walk around until that full feeling kicks in.

- Plan low-fat snacks for morning and afternoon (raw vegetables, breads, low-fat crackers).
- To avoid nibbling out of habit, choose two locations where you will eat all your food at home, and always sit down to eat.
- Eat slowly. Try to spend 25 minutes on each main meal.
- Avoid reading or watching TV while you are eating. Concentrate on your food, and enjoy it.
- Drink plenty of fluids (six to eight glasses each day).
- Start meals with a vegetable soup (without cream or excess sodium) or a salad with a low-fat or fat-free dressing. That will take the edge off your appetite.
- If you feel hungry when you think you shouldn't be, take a brisk walk or do some other type of workout. That will help take your mind off food and can actually reduce your appetite.

Dealing with Special Situations

Here are some common situations in which people overeat, and remedies you can try.

I often overeat when I'm in restaurants or with friends.   Some tips:

- Think ahead. Plan what you will say to refuse seconds.
- Plan to eat some low-fat food (such as bread) before you go, to cut your hunger pangs.
- Don't feel guilty if you leave food on the plate. In restaurants, ask for a doggy bag (especially if you have a dog).
- Be assertive in restaurants. Remember, you're paying, and you have a right to low-fat food. So ask for food the way *you* want it.

I eat when I'm under stress or depressed.   And when you've overeaten, you may still feel stressed or depressed. In fact, you might feel worse, because guilt is now mixed in with the other feelings. Some tips:

- Read the stress section, beginning on page 103.
- Practice instant relaxation, like this:

    Breathe in deeply while you count silently to five.
    Hold your breath while you count to five again.
    Breathe out slowly while you count to five.

As you breathe, let your abdomen expand—don't just breathe with your chest.

- When you feel stressed, change the scenery. Get up and go to another room, or walk around the block.
- Find a task that you've been putting off, and do it. (You'll feel good about yourself when you've finished.)
- Break the spell by talking to someone.

When I eat too much, I feel guilty about it and I stop trying to lose weight.   Remember, you are not "on a diet," so you can't "fall off" the diet. Sure, everyone eats too much sometimes. That's not important. What's important is the way you eat *most of the time*. If you ate more than you intended, don't be hard on yourself. Tell yourself that next time, you'll be better prepared for the situation that made you overeat. Simply start off again the next day with your low-fat way of eating.

STEP 6   KEEPING THE WEIGHT OFF

If you've lost weight before, you know that the hardest part can be keeping it off. And if you have tried to lose the weight through diet alone, without tuning up your body physically, the pounds you lost can come back much faster than you lost them. Why? Partly it's because you have lost muscle, which was your main calorie-consuming engine.

Also, when you weigh less, your body may simply need **less food.** Each pound of weight uses up about 11 to 12 calories a day, even when you don't exercise. When you lose pounds, you will need less food to stay at the same weight—unless you exercise. And it's almost impossible (and not very healthy) to live on the small amounts of food that would prevent you from gaining your weight back.

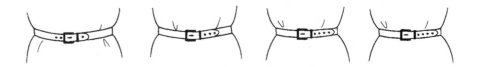

If you have tightened your belt a notch or two, congratulations! Your next challenge is to keep the buckle from moving back out again.

Here are some tips for keeping the weight off:

- When you've lost excess flab, don't think that you have finished the process. Think of it as a good start on a new way of living.
- If you find inches starting to come back, go back over the process again:

> Assess your exercise.
> Assess your fat intake.
> Get them back in balance.

It may be that even if you have cut your fat and increased your exercise considerably, your weight does not come down as much as you wanted. Perhaps it seems impossible to get it close to the ideal weight given in the "charts" for someone of your height and frame size.

But

> *If* you are looking after yourself in the way we describe in this book,
> *If* you are getting plenty of exercise,
> *If* you are eating a low-fat diet, with plenty of fruits and vegetables,
> *If* you do not have diabetes,
> *If* your blood pressure is under control and the doctor says your cholesterol levels are fine,
> And you *still* don't look like a model,

Don't worry about it. Maybe nature intended you to be larger than average. You can still be healthy, as long as you are eating a low-fat diet and getting your exercise.

Checking Up on Yourself

Remember, three months after you started the weight-loss program you should go back to Checkup No. 7 (on page 58). See how many minutes of activity you have added to your weekly routine.

And six months after you started the program, take Checkup No. 8 to see if it all worked!

Checkup No. 8   WHAT HAVE YOU LOST?

 Take this checkup six months after you started your flab-control program. See what changes you have made since you first answered these questions (see page 54):

Bend your arm. How much flesh can you pinch behind your upper arm?	____ A piece the size of my wrist ____ A piece the size of my thumb ____ A piece the size of my little finger
How much flesh can you pinch on your side, at the waistline, with your thumb on the top of the fold?	____ 2 inches or more ____ 1 to 2 inches ____ Less than 1 inch
Look at yourself in the mirror, and be honest. Are those bulges flab or muscle?	____ Pure flab ____ Half and half ____ Muscle
How much more do you weigh now than you did at age 20? (Skip this question if you were overweight then or if you are a serious body-builder who has added heavy muscles.)	____ 20 pounds or more ____ 10 to 20 pounds ____ Less than 10 pounds
Look at the belt you have worn for several years. In the last six months, did you have to move the buckle to a hole that made it longer? Or shorter?	____ I had to make it longer. ____ It's the same as it was. ____ It's shorter.
Would your spouse (or equivalent) still like you to lose weight?	____ Definitely ____ Probably ____ Not really

Exercise

If you started on the weight-control section before reading this, you may have already added some walking (or other exercise) to your daily routine. That's great. The more movement you can get into your life, the better. In this section, we help you to enjoy longer periods of exercise as you get into better physical shape, whether you are overweight or not.

This section has five steps:

1. Understand the benefits of exercise
2. Figure out how much exercise you get now
3. Begin a four-week walking program
4. Consider more vigorous forms of activity
5. See how far you have come

STEP 1 UNDERSTAND THE BENEFITS OF EXERCISE

Exercise can do several things:

- Regular exercise may lower blood pressure directly.
- It can help you reduce weight and keep it under control without starving yourself. (Marathon runners and long-distance bicyclists have no trouble staying thin.)
- It can help increase the "good" type of cholesterol in your blood and reduce the "bad" type (see "Your Cholesterol," page 14).
- It can provide you with the best natural tranquilizer, which in turn may help with your blood pressure (see the stress section, page 103).

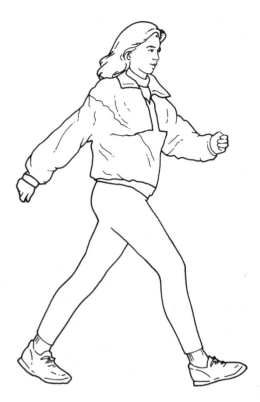

If exercise were a medicine, you probably wouldn't believe all the claims researchers make about it—even though they're true.

- It can get your heart and circulatory system into great shape. As your heart gets stronger, it will need fewer beats to do its work. This helps reduce the wear and tear on your blood vessels.
- For many people, it can become a healthy addiction. Exercise is something they positively enjoy. It can help counterbalance any feeling they may have of being deprived if they have to cut down on favorite foods or change other habits.
- Finally, exercise can give you more energy, make you feel good about yourself, and make you look better all over.

What Sort of Exercise Is Best?

The best exercise for making all of those improvements is the type that keeps your whole body moving at moderate speed—a speed that you can keep up for 20 minutes or more without stopping. Here are some examples:

Walking	Bicyling
Running	Swimming
Rowing	Skating
Dancing	Jumping rope
Jazzercise/aerobics	Skiing
Basketball	Soccer

This section of the book will get you started. But first, take Checkup No. 9.

STEP 2   FIGURE OUT HOW MUCH EXERCISE YOU GET NOW

First, here is a checkup to see where you are starting from.

FINDING YOUR STARTING POINT   Checkup No. 9

	Yes, More Than Once a Week	Sometimes, But Less Than Once a Week	No
Do you ever take walks in your spare time?			
Do you ever do other outdoor exercise (biking, running, etc.)?			
Do you play games that involve walking or running?			
Do you dance or do aerobics?			
Do you use machines (rowing, stair-stepping, treadmills, bikes, skiing)?			
Does your work ever involve walking for more than half an hour in a day?			

You will take this checkup again three months from now, to show how much more exercise you are doing. Meanwhile, there's one other little test: the pulse check.

Pulse Check

This is the way to take your resting pulse:

- Sit quietly for five minutes.
- Count your pulse at the wrist (on the same side as your thumb) or by pressing gently on your neck, one inch to either side of the windpipe (don't press hard enough to cut off the blood supply!).
- Count it for one minute.
- Repeat, later in the day. Write down the average of the two numbers here: _____.

In three months, you will do this test again to detect beneficial changes in your resting pulse rate. It should go down as you become fitter.

A Note about Safety

The first part of this exercise section is about walking. Walking (or swimming or bicycling) at moderate speed is safe for almost everyone and is excellent exercise. Check with your doctor if you have any doubts about whether these moderate forms of exercise are safe for you, or if you are concerned about a medical problem. Otherwise, go ahead.

Exercise that strains your body to the limit, such as weight lifting or sprinting, can raise blood pressure sharply. And strenuous exercise of any type (including vigorous biking and swimming or even fast walking) can be risky if you are not in good shape.

If you *do* want to do something vigorous, Step 4 of this section (starting on page 92) has a checkup for you, and plenty of advice on how to proceed safely. But don't skip to that section yet! We suggest you read through the information on walking first. Many of the tips for walkers are useful for everyone, and will help you set up a program of exercise you can stick to.

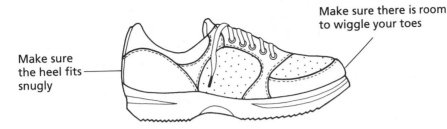

Make sure there is room
to wiggle your toes

Make sure
the heel fits
snugly

The great thing about walking is that it's free—except for the cost of shoes. And it's worth investing in a pair that will take you many miles.

STEP 3   BEGIN A FOUR-WEEK WALKING PROGRAM

Here's a four-week program to get you started on walking. Why, you may ask, do you need a program to help you do something you have been managing without much difficulty since the age of 1? For these reasons:

- The program will help you find time for walking.
- It will help you find ways to make it more entertaining.
- It will help you do it in a way that is useful.
- It will help you walk in a way that doesn't strain your muscles.
- It will help you overcome the reasons for *not* walking that might crowd into your head during the first weeks or months.

Week 1 of the Walking Program

Check off these steps as you take them:

_____ Think about shoes. If you don't have comfortable low-heeled shoes that have already taken you many miles, buy a pair of specialized walking or running shoes.
- Go to the largest (or best) sporting-shoe store in town, where the salespeople have plenty of experience. Don't rush. Tell the salesperson exactly what you want, and spend some time on your selection.
- Bring socks. Some people wear two pairs for serious walking—a thicker outer pair and a thinner pair next to the skin. But if the shoes fit well, one pair of socks should do.

- Make sure the shoes have a thick sole, support your heel, and give plenty of room to your toes.
- Don't buy until you have walked around the store in your shoes, making sure that your heel won't slide out, the shoes won't rub, and your toes have enough room.
- Look for sales—but don't go for the cheapest selection. Think of the shoes as an important investment in your health.

____ Plan the three times this week that you will walk for at least 15 minutes. Write them here:

Day	Time	Check When Done
1.		
2.		
3.		

Here are some thoughts to help you with the timing of walks:
- **Don't** walk at a time when the temperature is likely to be above 85 or 90 degrees.
- **Don't** walk right after meals. Wait two hours until the hard work of digestion is over and your body is ready for another challenge.
- **Do** walk before meals—especially if you want to lose weight. Believe it or not, moderate exercise can help take the edge off your appetite so that you are less likely to overeat.

____ If possible, arrange for someone to walk with you. Having another person involved can be helpful because you'll be less likely to change your mind at the last minute if someone is counting on you. And the walk will be more interesting.

____ Do it! Walk at the times you planned.
- Walk without carrying anything in your hands so that your arms can swing free. If you need to carry something, take along a fanny pack that you can wear around your waist.

- Always start slowly, then pick up the pace when your muscles have warmed up.
- Walk briskly, but don't let yourself get out of breath. If you find yourself breathing hard, slow down.

Week 2 of the Walking Program

The first task this week is to think about last week.

	Yes	No
Did you find time for the walks you had planned?		
Was your body comfortable?		
Did you enjoy the walks?		

If you have any checks in the "No" column, don't give up—spend a little more time planning this week's walks.

Finding Time to Walk   If finding time is a major problem, then consider one of these strategies:

- Combine walking with something else. If there's anyone you need to talk to, or want to talk to, do it on a walk. Use your walk to spend quality time with friends or family members (or the dog).
- Get up earlier. You may think that (a) getting less sleep and (b) starting off the day by doing something tiring would leave you in bad shape for the rest of the day. In fact, regular exercise can improve the quality of your sleep, so you won't miss the extra time in bed. And starting the day by walking can even give you more energy.
- Reconsider some of the other time-consuming things in your life, and see if you can make changes. For example, instead of watching the news on TV every night, take a walk—and listen to the news on a portable radio.

Was Your Body Uncomfortable?   If you had sore bones, joints, or muscles, slow down a little on your next walks. (And see page 99 for advice on prevention and treatment of minor injuries.)

- Check the warmup exercises on page 100, and start doing those stretches regularly. These exercises can help prevent injury and make your muscles more comfortable in their work.
- If your feet hurt, examine your shoes. Consider new ones. If they *are* new, adjust the socks and/or bandaids, and give them another chance.

Didn't You Enjoy the Walks?   If you didn't enjoy the walks, plan to pep them up:

- If you were bored, take along a person or a radio.
- If you didn't like the scenery, change it. Walk somewhere pretty.
- If the climate was terrible, go to the nearest heated or air-conditioned shopping mall, and walk around it briskly.
- Stick with it. Many people find walking becomes more pleasant as they get their mind and body into the right rhythm.

Tips for Climate Control

- In cold weather, pay attention to your head (wear a cap) and your hands (wear gloves). Wear light clothes in layers so that you can take off outer layers if and when you warm up.
- In hot weather, avoid the hottest times of the day. Wear light colors, and if you wear a hat to keep the sun off, get one that is well ventilated.

This Week's Plans   Plan for three walks of 20 to 25 minutes each:

Day	Time	Check When Done
1.		
2.		
3.		

This week, start thinking about the **way** you are walking.

Check off these steps after you take them:

_____ Swing your arms freely.

_____ Take along a watch. Count the number of strides per minute, and write the number here: _____.

_____ Try increasing the number of strides per minute by five. (If this makes you feel short of breath, drop back to your old pace. You can try to speed up again later, when you are in better shape.)

SAFETY NOTE: Any time you start breathing more deeply than usual when you are walking, take the "talk test." Talk to a friend, a dog, or yourself. If you are too short of breath to hold a conversation without strain—slow down your pace!

Week 3 of the Walking Program

First, take the same short checkup that you did last week.

	Yes	Yes and No	No
Did you find time for the walks you had planned?			
Was your body comfortable?			
Did you enjoy the walks?			

If You Checked "Yes"   Congratulations! You are on your way to becoming an addicted walker.

If You Checked "No"   At this point, "no" answers need to be taken seriously. If you are still not finding time for walks, still having aches and pains, and still not having a good time, then perhaps walking is not the best exercise for you.

   If you simply don't like walking much, it might be better to try some other form of moderate exercise, such as bicycling (outside or on

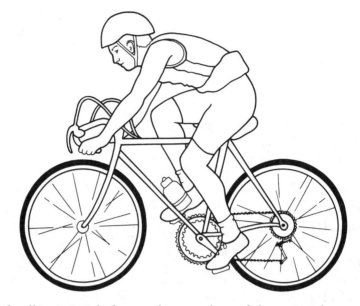

If walking isn't right for you, there are plenty of alternatives that can deliver moderate exercise—and even throw in some entertainment.

a machine). If you hurt, you might try swimming, which is much less hard on the joints. If you are bored, and you are in good shape, and your doctor approves, you might move on to the "vigorous activity" advice in Step 4 of this exercise section (page 92).

If You Checked "Yes and No"   You may still need to make some adjustments.

- Make sure that your shoes are giving you the support you need, without rubbing.
- Try walking on softer ground, like dirt or grass.
- Continue with the warmup stretches on page 100.
- Make an extra effort to find a time when you will not feel rushed or guilty; ask your family to help you.
- If taking walks just for the sake of walking isn't enjoyable, then try walking for a reason. For example, walk to work, or the library, or the store.

This Week's Plans   Make your week's plan for the three basic walks, which should now add up to 35 to 40 minutes each.

Day	Time	Check When Done
1.		
2.		
3.		

By now, you should be able to walk longer without feeling tired, and faster without getting breathless, but fitting in a walk of 35 to 40 minutes might be difficult. If necessary, split one or two of these walks into two. Walk to a mall 20 minutes away, then walk back. Or walk the last 20 minutes of your commute in the morning, and the first 20 minutes in the evening.

Recent research has shown that even if walks are split into smaller lengths of a few minutes at a time, you will still get the benefit. However, most people find it easier to keep track of their walking if they get it done in one or two sessions.

Week 4 of the Walking Program

From time to time, you may read about people who keep their good health until extreme old age—often whole populations, tucked away in remote corners of the world. You may hear different theories to explain the health and durability of these people, from wheat germ to yogurt, or strong systems of family support. But one important factor is this—these people tend to walk. They often walk many miles every day. And that could well be the secret of their long and healthy lives, because research in this country has also shown that people who walk live longer than people who don't.

Adding Time   Your three walks of 35 to 40 minutes each will have gone a long way toward improving your general health, and with it your blood pressure. But there's no need to stop there. Now that your legs are working well as a means of transportation, giving them more to do can produce added benefits.

This week, think of ways to fit additional walking into your routine. And just for the one week, use the blank form that follows to keep track of all walking that lasts longer than five minutes (including your long walks). See how high you can get your daily average. Walking an hour a day would be ideal, if you could find the time.

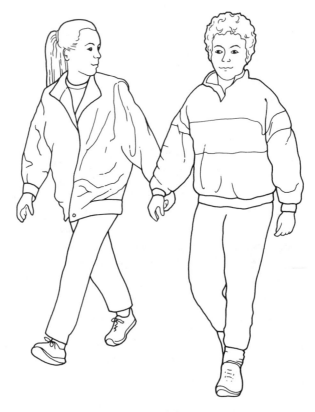

Walking adds years to your life and life to your years!

Keeping Track of Your Walks

Day	Time Spent	Where I Went	Daily Total
Sunday	1. _____ 2. _____ 3. _____ 4. _____	1. _____ 2. _____ 3. _____ 4. _____	 _____

Day	Time Spent	Where I Went	Daily Total
Monday	1. _____ 2. _____ 3. _____ 4. _____	1. _____ 2. _____ 3. _____ 4. _____	_____
Tuesday	1. _____ 2. _____ 3. _____ 4. _____	1. _____ 2. _____ 3. _____ 4. _____	_____
Wednesday	1. _____ 2. _____ 3. _____ 4. _____	1. _____ 2. _____ 3. _____ 4. _____	_____
Thursday	1. _____ 2. _____ 3. _____ 4. _____	1. _____ 2. _____ 3. _____ 4. _____	_____
Friday	1. _____ 2. _____ 3. _____ 4. _____	1. _____ 2. _____ 3. _____ 4. _____	_____
Saturday	1. _____ 2. _____ 3. _____ 4. _____	1. _____ 2. _____ 3. _____ 4. _____	_____

STEP 4 CONSIDER MORE VIGOROUS FORMS OF ACTIVITY

There is nothing wrong with sticking to walking for life. But some people prefer their exercise in a form that gets them into shape faster. Also, some people find other types of activity more fun.

In "What Sort of Exercise Is Best?" on page 80, we said that the best exercise for your blood pressure (and for your general health) is the type that keeps your whole body moving—especially your legs. A large number of activities fit into that category, some of them quite demanding and/or entertaining. Here are some advantages and disadvantages of the more adventurous types of activity.

Exercise Selection Chart

Activity	Comments
Jogging, running	If you are in good shape (see Checkup No. 10 on page 93), this can give you an excellent workout in a relatively short time. Be sure to follow the safety guidelines on pages 95–99. Jogging can be hard on feet, legs, hips, and back.
Vigorous walking	Walking fast, or uphill, or with a heavy backpack can be just as demanding as jogging and can get you into shape almost as fast. Some people do it carrying weights for upper-body strengthening.
Bicycling	An advantage of bicycling is that your weight is supported, so it is easy on the joints and is particularly suited to people with arthritis.
Swimming	Slow swimming is great for flexibility but does not give you much of a workout. Moderate or fast swimming can be excellent for conditioning.
Roller skating	If you are padded to avoid the risk of major injuries (which are all too common), in-line skates provide wonderful exercise and a good deal of entertainment (both to you and, perhaps, to spectators).
Ice skating	If there's ice available, this is excellent exercise.

Activity	Comments
Skiing	Cross-country skiing (on snow or on a machine) can be one of the most demanding and effective forms of exercise.
Rowing	Rowing (whether on a lake or a machine) can give you a good workout for the whole body, if you do it right.
Dancing, jazzercise, or aerobics	Moving to music is one way of making exercise enjoyable, whether with a partner or in a class. The advantage of classes is that a trained instructor will help you stay at the most appropriate level and help you avoid aches and pains.
Tennis	Singles tennis can give you a good workout; doubles may have too much stopping, starting, and waiting for your partner to get the ball over the net.
Basketball, squash, racquetball, soccer	These games are only for the very fit—and if you qualify (see Checkup No. 10), they can make you fitter in a hurry.

Are You in Shape?

As we said on page 82, people who want to take up an activity that is more vigorous than moderate-speed walking, bicycling, or swimming should make sure they are in good enough condition. Here's a checkup to help you decide.

YOUR PHYSICAL CONDITION   Checkup No. 10

	YES	NO
WEIGHT *Are you within 20 pounds of what you weighed (or wanted to weigh) at age 20?*		

	YES	NO
BLOOD PRESSURE *Is your blood pressure either borderline (see page 9) or lower?*		
HEART DISEASE *As far as you know, are you free of heart disease? Are you free of recurrent chest pains?*		
OTHER MEDICAL CONDITIONS *Are you free of chronic medical conditions for which you see the doctor regularly?*		
AGE *(see safety note on next page)* *Are you under 45?*		

Or:

PHYSICAL CONDITION *Have you been doing one of the vigorous types of exercise on page 92 regularly, without any problems?*		

Or:

MEDICAL CLEARANCE *Has your doctor specifically cleared you for vigorous exercise?*		

Checking with Your Doctor   If you can't answer "Yes" to all the questions in Checkup No. 10, it is best to talk to the doctor before you take up a vigorous form of exercise. If you are relatively young and have no problems besides your raised blood pressure—and that's under control—your doctor probably will tell you that it's safe to start some form of exercise that's more demanding than walking on level ground (as long as you follow safety guidelines like those on pages 95–99). If there is any doubt about whether you're in good enough shape for vigorous exercise, you may be given a "stress EKG," which involves walking on a treadmill while your heart is monitored.

Safety in Middle Age   If you are a fit 47- or even 57-year-old, you may wonder whether you really need to check with your doctor before breaking into a jog. The answer depends partly on your own circumstances. The problem is that fitness doesn't "keep," so even if you were in great shape the year before last, it won't help much now. If you don't use it, you lose it, and have to start building it up again from scratch.

And risk does increase with age. A young adult may survive sudden strains that someone of middle age may not. So talk to your doctor if you are over 45 and want to *start* vigorous exercise *unless*:

- You've been exercising at a moderate level continuously, without any problems—for example, brisk walks at least three times a week;
- You intend to add more vigorous activity very gradually—for example, starting with one minute of slow jogging for every three minutes of walking;
- *And* you will follow all the safety guidelines—for example, using your heart rate as a guide (see page 97).

SAFETY GUIDELINES

There are two main ways to make sure you are not straining your heart or other vital parts:

1. Use your heart rate as a monitor.
2. Use common sense.

And remember, it can take a couple of months to get up to speed if you haven't been exercising regularly (longer if you want to race). So don't try to do too much too soon.

The Heart Rate

When your large muscles are working hard, they need extra oxygen, and your heart speeds up to pump more oxygen-rich blood to the parts that need it. This extra work strengthens your heart and tones up the whole circulatory system.

How fast should your heart beat? We will give you a heart-rate "target range" for someone of your age. This will help you avoid straining your heart, and it will tell you whether you are exercising hard enough to do your heart and circulatory system (including blood pressure) some good.

- If your heart is going faster than the safe range for your age, you should slow down.
- If your heart is not going as fast as the range for your age, you are not getting all the benefit from exercise that you could, and you can exercise more vigorously.

Finding Your Pulse   Practice finding your pulse and counting it for a minute. Most people use the pulse at their wrist to find their heart rate, but you can also check it on your neck, about an inch to either side of the windpipe. Remember not to press the artery in your neck too hard while you count (cutting off the supply of blood to your brain is not a good idea).

Finding the Target Rate   Your heart has a **maximum** speed that depends on your age. It should not—repeat, not—ever go that fast. For now, your safe target heart rate for exercise will be a percentage of the maximum, between 65% and 75%. (Later, when you are running marathons, it can go higher.)

There are two ways to find this safe target rate—one complicated and one simple:

Complicated
Subtract your age from 220. That's your maximum heart rate. Then calculate 65% to 75% of that. That's your safe target rate.

Simple
Use the table below to find the figure for your age group. As you get closer to the next age category, adjust your heart beat downward.

TARGET HEART-RATE RANGE FOR DIFFERENT AGES
65%–75% maximum capacity (beats per minute)

Age	20	30	40	50	60	Over 70
Range	130–150	123–142	117–135	110–127	104–120	97–112

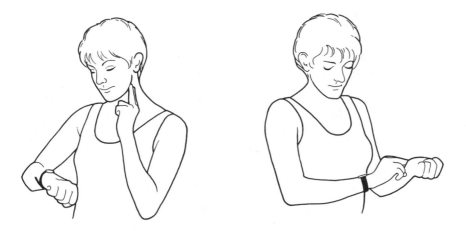

You have a built-in monitor that helps you exercise hard enough, but not too hard: your pulse.

Here's the target range for 10 seconds:

Age	20	30	40	50	60	Over 70
Range	23–25	22–24	21–23	19–21	18–20	17–19

In the beginning, you may need to check your pulse quite often to see that your heart-rate is within the target range for your age.

- Check it now, for practice.
- Check it when you have been exercising for 5 minutes.
- Check it again every 10 minutes or so while you are exercising, or if you have a hunch it has gone up (or down).

Using Common Sense

Common sense can be just as important as numbers in helping you to exercise safely.

- Always start exercising *slowly*, and let all your working parts (including your heart) ease into the session gradually.

- If you feel weak or dizzy, or have a pain in your chest, slow down (and tell your doctor).
- Take the "talk test." Don't let yourself get so breathless that you can't hold a conversation.
- Monitor your "RPE." That stands for "rate of perceived exertion." In other words, how hard do you *think* your body is working? If it seems too hard, slow down. If you have a suspicion that you are not going fast enough to do any good, speed up (but check your heart rate).
- **Don't** exercise when the temperature is over 90 degrees.
- **Don't** exercise right after a meal. Wait two hours.
- **Do** make sure you drink plenty of water in hot weather—before, after, and (if necessary) during exercise. There's no need for fancy sport drinks—plain water is best.
- **Don't** do vigorous exercise if you have a cold or fever.
- **Do** exercise regularly. The benefits can't be stored—you need to keep doing it.
- If you have to stop exercise for a week or more for any reason, start again slowly.

WARM-UPS AND COOL-DOWNS

When you start a vigorous exercise program, you are likely to use muscles and tendons that have been comfortably asleep for years. In some cases, if you try to do too much too fast, there is a risk of injury. In other cases, there is merely the likelihood of aches and pains. Your working body parts may feel quite sore if you surprise them with a workload they hadn't expected.

Warm-ups

Warm-ups can help you make working muscles flexible and reduce the chance of injury. They come in two types:

1. *Warm-ups for the whole body.* You do these by starting your exercise slowly. For example:

> Do a few slow lengths of the pool before you build up to your
>   regular swimming speed;
> Start a run with a mixture of walking and slow jogging;
> Pedal the bike slowly for the first few minutes.

2. *Warm-ups for the separate parts.* These exercises stretch your muscles
   to help get them ready, and to help prevent injury (see page 100).

Cool-downs

Cool-downs are not as important as warm-ups in preventing injury,
but they can help you avoid unpleasant surprises. At the end of vigorous
activity, your circulation slows down, leaving more blood in your legs
(where it was needed) than in your brain. The cool-down period helps your
circulation to even out so that your brain gets its fair share again. Without
a cool-down, you might feel faint. It's not complicated: Just walk around
slowly for a few minutes when the vigorous part of your workout is over.
Or swim slowly, or pedal slowly.

Some people repeat the warm-up exercises on page 100 at this time,
because their muscles are still soft and pliable and the exercises are easier.

INJURIES

If you get aches and pains, apply some ice for 10 minutes or so, take an
aspirin or equivalent for the inflammation, and, if necessary, slow down
during your next exercise session.

For more serious strains or sprains, including those that need to be
checked out by a doctor, you probably will be advised to use the **RICE**
treatment:

Rest the part.
Ice it, for 15 to 20 minutes at a time.
Compress it, by wrapping in an elastic bandage.
Elevate it; keep the part raised up so that blood doesn't collect in it.

WARM-UP

Spend one or two minutes on each exercise. Do them slowly, with no bouncing. And if anything hurts—back off.

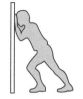

WALL STRETCH
Stand about 3 feet from a wall. Lean forward, with your hands against the wall at shoulder height (don't bend at the waist). Put one foot forward keeping both heels on the floor and the back leg straight. Lean in slowly towards the wall, and hold the stretch for 10–20 seconds. Repeat 3 times with each leg.

HAMSTRING STRETCH
Put one foot on a curb, car fender, or something else at a comfortable height, toe pointing upwards and leg straight. Bend the other knee slightly and lean forward at the hips, keeping head up and back straight. Hold a moment then switch legs.

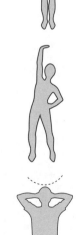

QUADRICEP STRETCH
Balance on your left leg with your left arm up, thumb back. With your right hand, hold your right foot. Gently push it into your hand, and hold. Repeat with left foot. (If you can't balance, hold on to something.)

ARM CIRCLES
Hold your arms straight out. Draw a circle about one foot across with both hands at once. Repeat five times in each direction.

SIDE STRETCH
Stand with your feet 18 inches apart, hips centered. Raise one hand, palm upwards, fingers pointing inwards. Stand straight, or bend just a few inches. Feel the stretch in your side. Repeat with other arm raised.

NECK STRETCH
Clasp hands behind your neck, and look along your left shoulder. Slowly tilt your head down and to the front, as you look at your toes. Then continue the movement smoothly until you are looking along your right shoulder. Don't tilt your head back.

Time spent stretching out your tendons and muscles will pay off—in a greatly reduced risk of injury.

STEP 5 SEE HOW FAR YOU HAVE COME

Three months after you have started, re-take the checkup from page **81**

YOUR THREE-MONTHS PROGRESS CHART   Checkup No. 11

	Yes, More Than Once a Week	Sometimes, But Less Than Once a Week	No
Do you take walks in your spare time?			
Do you ever do other outdoor exercise (biking, running, etc.)?			
Do you play games that involve walking or running?			
Do you dance or do aerobics?			
Do you use machines (rowing, stair-stepping, treadmills, bikes, skiing)?			
Does your work ever involve walking for more than half an hour in a day?			

Now answer the following questions:

	Yes	No
Do you feel stronger?		
Do you feel more energetic?		
Do people say you look better?		
Do you find that you miss exercise when you don't do it?		

Now find your resting heart rate, and see if it has gone down.

- Sit quietly for five minutes.
- Count your pulse.
- Write down the average of the two numbers: _____.

CONCLUSION

It is said that the hardest part of any exercise program is getting your foot outside the door (or on to a machine, if you use exercise machines at home). If you have overcome all the excuses that your brain may have cooked up to keep you from getting your foot outside the door (or on to the machine)—congratulations. After three months, your body is probably starting to positively want its exercise, and may even demand it!

Here are two brief reminders:

- Exercise can't be stored. You need to keep it up regularly to get the benefits.
- If you stop for any reason, you may get out of condition depressingly fast. So when you start again, you may have to build up your stamina gradually, almost as if you were a beginner.

But here's the good news: If you have managed to get into the habit of regular exercise, you have taken one of the most important steps toward improving the *quality* of your life, as well as your health. And your blood pressure will show the difference.

Stress

Almost everyone is under stress sometimes, and it's certainly not always harmful. People with jobs that seem to be full of stress (such as orchestra conductors) often live into very old age. The excitement of their work seems to keep them young and lively.

However, certain kinds of stress can be harmful. In this section, we will help you to identify what causes *your* stress, and to decide whether that level of stress could be affecting your blood pressure and your general health. And we'll help you find ways to calm down, if you need to.

HOW DAMAGING IS STRESS?

It's popular to blame stress for high blood pressure, as well as other problems. Imagine the high-powered executive roaring at his subordinates, red in the face, veins bulging. Probably many of us would suspect he suffers from high blood pressure. But this type of stress may not affect blood pressure seriously at all. As soon as the boss has stopped yelling, his pressure may go down again.

There has been a great deal of research recently about the harmfulness of stress, and the verdict is mixed. The general conclusion is that *frequent* stress is not healthful for those with high blood pressure—partly because of the way it temporarily boosts pressure, and partly because people who are under stress may find it hard to look after themselves. They often tend to eat, smoke, or drink too much, and don't find time for exercise.

So the bottom line is this: If you have high blood pressure, you would be wise to find ways to bring your stress level down. But don't reach a point where you are so worried about stress that you develop more stress. For most people, stress control will be less important to their blood pressure than the factors addressed earlier in this book, such as sodium reduction and weight control.

THE VALUE OF STRESS

Stress was very useful for prehistoric people, and helped them survive. It gave them the strength they needed to fight bears, run away from wolves, or get out of the way of falling rocks. And when modern people are under severe stress, their body instantly produces hormones that get them ready for the same type of physical "fight or flight":

- Your blood vessels clamp down to direct blood to your brain and to the muscles that you need to run or fight.
- Your heart speeds up, to get more oxygen to your brain and muscles.
- Your digestion stops so that it won't use up energy that's needed elsewhere.
- Your muscles get a burst of strength.

This system works fine when the stressful situation requires you to do something physical, like running from a mugger or lifting a car off someone's leg. It doesn't work well in the situations that are most likely to cause us stress in modern life. For example:

You are not supposed to run away from a boss who is criticizing your work.
You are not supposed to hit the foreman who is yelling in your face.
Your extra physical energy won't speed up the checkout line or help you cope with difficult teenagers.

Yet those stress hormones still flood your system, preparing you for action. And if you are under stress frequently, this can harm your physical health.

WHAT CAUSES YOU STRESS?

Each person will have a different list of stressful situations, because events affect people in different ways. *You* might hate standing in line, while your

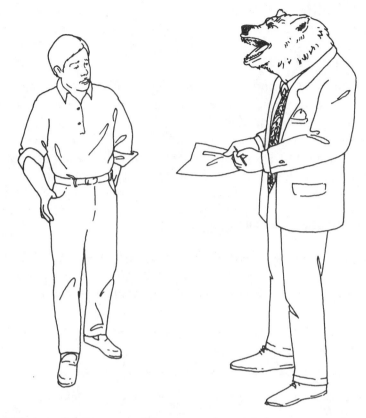

"Flight or fight" was a useful response when early humans came face to face with wild animals. It may not work quite so well in the modern workplace.

spouse doesn't mind a bit. *You* might grind your teeth with tension in a situation that your co-worker merely finds challenging. There are certain situations, however, that experts agree are likely to increase everyone's stress levels: life changes, lack of control, and poor communication.

Life Changes

You are more likely to be under stress at times when major changes are under way, whether they are "good" or "bad." A new job, a new baby, a child's wedding, a death, a divorce, moving to a new community—all of these are stressful situations.

Lack of Control

You are more likely to be under stress if you can't control the amount of work coming your way.

> A waitress who cannot limit the number of customers she has to serve may be under more stress than one who knows she can get help if the workload reaches a certain point.
>
> Assembly-line workers may be highly stressed if someone else controls the speed of the line. If they have the power to regulate the speed themselves, much of the stress will evaporate.

Poor Communication

You may be under stress if you can't express your own needs clearly. Or you may put people's backs up because you seem much more aggressive than you intend. They may overreact—and the result is more stress for you.

DEALING WITH YOUR OWN STRESS

In this section, we will take you through four steps:

1. Identify your stress
2. Keep track of your stress
3. Learn to deal with stressful situations
4. Practice stress-proofing your body (and mind)

STEP 1 IDENTIFY YOUR STRESS

Stress can show up in a number of different ways: in your body, your emotions, or your habits. Here's a checkup for different symptoms of stress that you may experience.

WHAT ARE YOUR SYMPTOMS?   Checkup No. 12

1. Physical signs of stress

Do you have any of the following symptoms at times when you feel tense?

Symptom	Yes	No	Sometimes
Headaches			
Stomach upset			
Tension in muscles (sore neck or back)			
Grinding your teeth			
Sweating			
Trouble sleeping			
Fatigue			
Lack of appetite			

2. Emotional signs of stress

Does stress show up often in your moods?

Symptom	Yes	No	Sometimes
Do you often feel nervous?			
Do you easily get sad or depressed?			
Do you often get angry and hostile?			
Do you feel suspicious of the world around you?			
Do you feel panicked because you are afraid you won't get things done on time?			

3. Habits

Sometimes stress shows up in the way people act:

Symptom	Yes	No	Sometimes
Do you eat or drink too much when you are under stress?			
If you smoke, do you think it is because you are under stress?			

The more "Yes" answers you checked, the greater your stress level is likely to be. You may or may not have a stressful way of life—but your mind and your body act as if you do. And that's what is most important.

STEP 2 KEEP TRACK OF YOUR STRESS

In this step, you will practice identifying **stressors**—the circumstances (or people) that cause *you* stress. Notice that the emphasis is on "you." These stressors may not cause other people stress—they are your own personal property. Remember, something that one person finds stressful might present no problems for someone else.

First, you will keep a stress diary, recording everything that causes you stress for a couple of days.

The "Stress Diary"

Look through the symptoms of stress that you checked in Checkup No. 12. Then make a note if you experience one of those symptoms, whether it's a physical one, such as tooth-grinding or muscle tension, or an emotional one, like feelings of anxiety. Also note when you feel the need to eat, smoke, or drink because you are under stress.

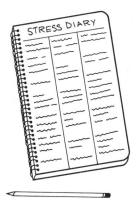

The first step towards reducing stress is to recognize when you have it—and keep track of it.

Here's a sample:

Day	Time	What I Felt or Did	What Was Happening
Monday	8 a.m.	Stomach muscles tight; headache starting	Stuck in traffic
	8:20	Depressed	Dan said I have to do my report over
	10	Ate two donuts	Argument with Jen about window

If you can't bring out your notebook and make a full entry at the time you notice the symptom of stress, write a word or two about it on any piece of paper, and make a complete entry when you have time.

Using Your Diary

After two days, study your list and look for patterns.

- Decide which of your stressful moments were caused by some **external** factor, such as money problems, health problems, time problems, or demands on you at work.

- Then decide which were **internal,** caused mostly by your difficulty in communicating, or anxiety about things that are not really very important, or your competitive feelings, or the fact that you demand perfection of yourself and others.

Sometimes it helps to list your stressors like this:

Stuck in traffic:	External
Mad at Dan:	External (he's an **$#*) and internal (I overreacted)
Anxious about kids:	Internal—no real reason to worry

What Are Your Main Stressors?

When you have had some practice in thinking about the causes of stress in your life, take the following checkup to help you realize what's bugging you, and what most needs attention.

Checkup No. 13   IDENTIFYING YOUR OWN STRESSORS

 Check stressors that you have and add any others you may have.

1. External Stressors	A major problem	A moderate problem	I can live with it
A life change is affecting you (such as a new job, new baby).			
There's not enough time to get everything done.			
People at work are giving you a hard time (and you are not imagining this).			
You are worried about money or health.			
Other:			
Other:			
Other:			

2. Internal Stressors	A major problem	A moderate problem	I can live with it
You are having trouble communicating with family members or co-workers.			
You are having trouble organizing your day.			
You feel competitive.			
You have aggressive feelings.			
You have problems with depression and self-esteem.			
You are worried about events in your community or the world.			
Other:			
Other:			
Other:			

Later, we will give you suggestions for working on some of these problems. Meanwhile, here are some "first aid" tips you can use to lower your level of stress any time it feels too high for comfort.

First Aid for Stress

On the next page you will find different remedies that work for different people. Check those you've tried, and then check the ones that seem best for you.

Try one of these remedies the next time you feel stressed out:	Check if you've tried this.	Check if it works for you.
Count to ten.		
Practice deep breathing. Relax, then breathe so that your whole abdomen goes in and out—not just your chest. Breathe in slowly, while you count to five under your breath. Hold your breath while you count to five again, then breathe out slowly, once more counting to five.		
Order your muscles to relax.		
Take a walk around the block.		
Move to a different room in the house or your workplace, even if it just means going down the hall to the bathroom.		
Change what you are doing. Distract yourself by switching to a different task, or picking up a newspaper or magazine, or changing the channel on the radio or TV.		
Talk to someone. It doesn't have to be about what's troubling you—any conversation can help break the spell.		
Drink a glass of water or juice.		
Find something low-calorie to eat or chew.		
Find a safe place for your mind. Switch it to memories of a good vacation, or plans for the weekend.		
Hug someone (or the dog).		

STEP 3   LEARN TO DEAL WITH STRESSFUL SITUATIONS

In this step, we help you to develop some long-term solutions to some of the problems you identified in Steps 1 and 2. But keep in mind that there's a limit to what can be done through a self-help program like this. If you are seriously stressed, and none of the "home remedies" we suggest make much of a dent in your stress levels, then you may need more help. For example, you could check into the stress-reduction programs offered by a local YMCA, hospital, clinic, community college, or mental health agency. If you decide that stress and anger are a serious health problem for you, you may want to see a counselor (your doctor should be able to help with this decision).

If your problems are not too serious, the following suggestions should help.

Managing Your Time

Better time management can be helpful, whether you really have too much to do or are simply bad at organizing the tasks you have. By giving structure to your day, time management can also relieve the stress that can come from boredom.

- Make a plan for the day. It's best to write it down, though some people just form plans in their head. Make sure to allow time for the things that must get done.

- Set aside times to deal with routine tasks, like telephoning or answering the mail, so that you can get them out of the way.

- Leave some time for yourself—for example, plan time for a walk or reading for pleasure.

- Don't plan the day to be absolutely full. Leave some spare time to cope with any emergencies or to allow for the fact that certain tasks may take longer than you expected. And you may want to allow time just in case something comes up that you really want to do.

- To save time, plan to do two things at once. For example, read important material while you are on your exercise bicycle; combine errands; encourage the family to eat together so that you can discuss any family business at meal times.

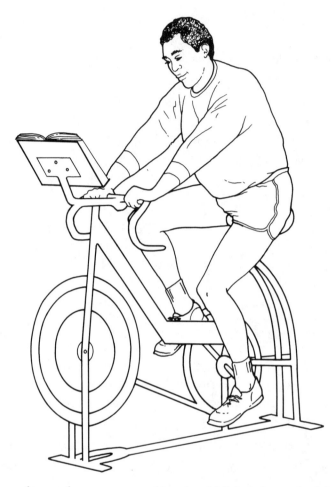

Is your day too short to get everything done? Make it longer by doing two things at once.

- Delegate. Get others at work or in the family to take over some of your tasks (or do their fair share).

Communicating Better

As you looked over your stress diary, you may have thought, "I should have said . . ." or "He didn't understand. . . ."

Better communication can often take the stress out of situations—but it's not always easy. You may find it hard to state your point of view (being assertive) without coming on too strong (being aggressive). It needs practice. Here are some tips:

- Try to anticipate when difficult situations are coming up, and practice what you will say.
- State your point of view, without blaming anyone else. (Not "You never give me enough time," but "I really need a little more time.")
- Listen! Concentrate on what the other person has to say.
- Make absolutely sure you both understand what's going on. For example, say, "Let's see if I've got this right. What you are saying is. . . ."
- Try to get the other person to agree to a plan that helps avoid conflict in the future.
- If you are about to explode, take a time out. You may have heard that it is better to express your anger than to bottle it up—but often putting angry thoughts into words will make things worse. It's better to move away from the situation or change the subject. Take up the topic when you are calm enough to discuss it.
- Don't let people walk all over you (and spend the rest of the day fuming about it). Speak up. For example, if someone has done a sloppy home-repair job for you, calmly point out what is wrong.

Changing Your Thoughts

You may think it is hard to change what's going on in your head, but try it. It often works.

- When a stressful thought turns up in your head (for example, you find yourself thinking that you are going to fail or be in trouble), stop it. Simply say, "Stop!"
- If you are tense because you are brooding about something, make an effort to change the subject of your thoughts. Move to a different room; turn on the radio or TV; or telephone someone. Think about children, or grandchildren, or your favorite team (if they are doing well) or your next vacation.

Dealing with Problem Situations

Here are three ways you can approach situations that often cause you stress:

- **Avoid** the situation. For example, if you often panic about getting stuck in traffic on the way to work, try a different type of commute, or work flex-time to avoid the rush hour.
- **Adapt** to the situation. For example, if you get tense standing in line, make a point of always carrying a book with you.
- **Alter** the situation. For example, if you've been having trouble finishing work on time, get together with your boss or co-workers. Agree on a new system that helps you get things done.

Sometimes, you may feel physically tense even when there is no apparent reason for it. The next step may help you to reduce this type of stress.

STEP 4   PRACTICE STRESS-PROOFING YOUR BODY (AND MIND)

In this step, we will help you to make your body feel more relaxed.

Some people get into the habit of living with a high level of physical tension. They can't sit still, their muscles tend to be tense—and this can keep their blood pressure high. Learning to relax may not be enough on its own to bring pressure down, but it can help.

We will tell you about the four ways you can get your body to calm down: through exercise, better quality sleep, cutting down on chemicals, and deep muscle relaxation.

Get Regular Exercise

We hope you are getting regular exercise already. If not, try it, following the suggestions in the exercise section. Exercise can help in a number of ways:

- It gives you a time out from your routine and a change of scenery.
- It makes you feel good about what you are doing for yourself.
- Sustained, vigorous exercise (like walking very briskly for a half hour or running for 20 minutes or so) can act as a tranquilizer. It makes you feel good all over.

Check Up on Your Sleep Patterns

One of the best ways to sleep badly is to worry about sleeping badly. Not everyone needs a full eight hours—and the quality of your sleep may be as important as its length. However, if you *frequently* have trouble getting to sleep, or if you wake up early or often, and if you feel sleepy or irritable during the day, here are some suggestions:

- Consider how much caffeine you are getting, in cola, coffee, and tea. Try cutting it out late in the day, or even all the time.
- Get more exercise, which will give you a healthy sort of tiredness. But don't exercise late in the day: The short-term effect may be to make you feel alert.
- Go to bed at about the same time each night.
- If you have naps, keep them to 20 minutes or less.
- Don't make yourself sleepy with alcohol or sleeping drugs. They will interfere with the *quality* of your sleep so that even if you succeed in keeping your eyes shut for longer, you won't wake up refreshed.
- If you still have frequent trouble sleeping (more than once or twice a month), talk to your doctor.

Watch the Chemicals

In the next section of this book, we'll talk about possible effects of caffeine and alcohol on your blood pressure. For now, think about their effects on your stress levels.

- Does caffeine speed you up? Try cutting down. (See page 122 for suggestions.)
- Are you in the habit of taking more than two alcoholic drinks a day? That amount of alcohol can start to mess up your moods (and can also raise your blood pressure). You may feel that a drink relieves stress—but the long-term effects may be the opposite.
- Do you smoke to relax yourself? Forget it—nicotine is a stimulant. In fact, one of the main problems that people report when they quit is that they feel sleepy. (See the next section for suggestions on how to quit.)

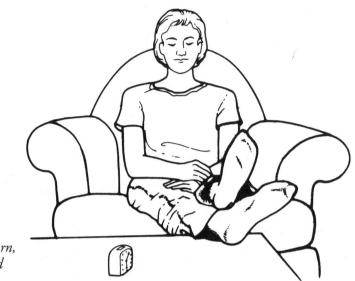

Deep relaxation is not hard to learn, and it can pay off in less stress and lower blood pressure.

Learn Deep Relaxation

Regular relaxation can help to "stress-proof" you and turn you into a calmer person. Here's one method that has even been shown to work on reducing blood pressure levels:

1. Set aside 15 minutes for relaxing at least two or three times a week.
2. Find a comfortable chair in a room where you can be completely alone.
3. Set an alarm for 15 minutes so that you won't need to worry about the time.
4. Sit down and close your eyes. Then relax each group of muscles in the order below, until every part of you feels floppy and warm. Sometimes it helps to tighten up the muscles before you relax them so that you can feel the contrast. Start with your **right arm,** then go around in this order:

(1) Right thigh	(6) Abdomen and buttocks
(2) Right calf	(7) Diaphragm and chest
(3) Right ankle and foot	(8) Neck
(4) Left leg (thigh, calf, foot)	(9) Jaw
(5) Left arm	(10) Forehead

5. When your whole body is completely relaxed, empty your mind. Think of a soothing scene, like ripples on a lake shore, or soft breezes wafting through grass.
6. After the alarm goes off, sit quietly for a few more minutes, while you adjust to reality.

CONCLUSION

Stress is hard to measure, so it may be difficult to judge whether or not you have managed to reduce it. One way of keeping track is to keep a stress diary for a couple of days every month. This will tell you what still needs attention—and also whether your stress-reduction measures are working, gradually, to take the most unpleasant aspects of stress from your life.

Fine-tuning Your Life

No matter how carefully you improve your way of living by eating right and getting your body into shape, your efforts may be wasted if you are raising your blood pressure with chemicals. Street drugs like cocaine have a direct effect on blood pressure—but so also do legal drugs, such as alcohol, nicotine, and, for some people, caffeine.

ALCOHOL

You may have heard that moderate alcohol intake can help reduce the risk of heart disease. It's true that one or two drinks a day can increase the beneficial type of cholesterol in your blood (high density lipoprotein, or HDL). But the disadvantages of alcohol can easily outweigh any advantage. If you take more than a couple of drinks a day, the net effect will be harmful to your heart, as well as your liver and other organs. For some people, two or more drinks a day also increase blood pressure.

Here are some tips for those who may need to cut down:

- If you don't want to stop drinking altogether, aim to cut down to two drinks or less a day.
- Drink only with meals.
- If you expect to be in situations where you might be tempted to drink too much, plan ahead. Have a nonalcoholic drink between alcoholic drinks. Take drinks in tall glasses (beer, or wine with soda) and sip to make them last longer.
- If it is hard to cut down to two drinks a day, consider quitting altogether. It will be easier in the long run.

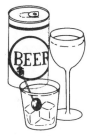

A shot of liquor, a glass of wine, a can of beer—whatever you drink, it's all the same to your blood pressure. More than one or two drinks a day can be harmful.

NICOTINE

Cigarettes kill many more people through heart disease and stroke than through cancer:

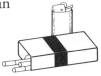

- They speed up the clogging of the arteries.
- They speed up the action of the heart, and constrict blood vessels, which can push up blood pressure.
- They can make the heartbeat irregular, which can be dangerous.

More than 40 million Americans have quit smoking.

Think of people you know who died of heart attacks or strokes before they reached 50, or even 60. How many of them smoked? Probably most of them. For people with high blood pressure, smoking is especially dangerous.

If you smoke, you probably mean to quit. The question is, how? If you have tried already and didn't make it, you may not feel good about your chances. However, millions have quit, and most had to try more than once before they were cigarette-free for life. Here are some suggestions:

- Talk to your doctor about using the nicotine patch. He or she will consider your blood pressure levels and general state of health when deciding whether or not to prescribe it. The patch can be useful in helping smokers overcome the physical dependence on nicotine during the early weeks.
- Whether you are using the patch or not, follow these suggestions:

  Set a date for quitting.
  Prepare substitutes (low-calorie foods; treats that give you pleasure; activities to distract you).

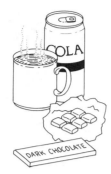

Of all the addictive drugs, caffeine is perhaps the most harmless—but it's a bad idea to overdose.

Plan ahead for any situations that you feel may tempt you to smoke. Avoid those situations, or prepare for them by planning what you will say or do to defend yourself against temptation.

When a craving hits, move! Walk to another room. Do something. Take a drink of water. Talk to a friend. Look at your watch—the cravings will get shorter as the days go by.

Breathe deeply. Breathe in slowly while you count silently to five. Hold your breath while you count to five again. Breathe out on the count of five.

- Expect to go through some rough times during the first weeks—but keep telling yourself it's worth it. Talk to people who have already quit. They will assure you that you are doing one of the best things you possibly could for your health.

- Tell yourself that you don't have a choice. If your blood pressure is high, quitting is essential.

CAFFEINE

Caffeine need not be harmful. Even though it may boost blood pressure temporarily, the pressure doesn't stay high. However, some doctors will suggest that their patients drink less coffee—particularly if it is interfering with sleep or making it hard to relax. As a rule of thumb, it's smart to cut down if you are drinking more than two strong cups a day.

Caffeine is an addictive drug. If you cut it out completely, you may have withdrawal symptoms for a few days, including sleepiness and a dull headache. To help avoid such symptoms, try cutting down gradually:

- Each week, switch one of your daily cups of coffee to a decaffeinated type. Finally, switch over completely to decaf.
- Explore the many tastes of herbal teas.
- Switch from caffeinated colas to soft drinks without caffeine or (better) to water or juice.

How Far Have You Come?

If you have worked through this book, and taken some (or even all) of its advice, how are you doing? Here is another copy of the checkup that you first met at the beginning of the book, on page 24. Take the checkup again, to see if your "risk score" has changed.

MEASURE YOUR PROGRESS Checkup No. 14

Remember, there's one factor you can't do anything about:

Family *Give yourself one point if a parent, brother, or sister had (or has) high blood pressure.*	

Next, here are the five factors you can control:

Weight *Pinch the flesh at the side of your waist (thumb on top of the fold). Give yourself one point for each inch you can pinch.*	

Salt *If you salt food at the table, give yourself one point.* *If you often eat salty snacks like chips, nuts, or pretzels, give yourself another point.* *If you use prepared foods like frozen dishes, soups, sauces, or mixes (and don't pick low-sodium types), or often eat out at fast-food restaurants, give yourself one more point.*	
Exercise *If you don't walk (or do other exercise) three or four days a week for at least 20 minutes on each of those days, that's one point. If you are a real couch potato, two points.*	
Stress *If you feel uncomfortably stressed more than once a day, give yourself a point.*	
Chemicals *A little coffee or alcohol probably won't affect your blood pressure, but if you think that you are revving up your motor with too much caffeine, alcohol, or other drugs, give yourself a point.*	
Total	

TROUBLESHOOTING

If you have not yet brought down your risk score as far as you would like, spend some extra time going over the sections of the book that can help. For example, if your weight is still not where you'd like it, reread that section. If necessary, cut out more fat or get more exercise. Or perhaps just be patient—you may need more time.

If your risk score has come down because you are doing everything right, but your blood pressure has not, talk to your doctor. He or she will urge you to keep up with your new way of living and may simply tell you to be patient. Or you may need additional help in the form of medication.

FOR THE FUTURE . . .

If you have brought down your blood pressure, congratulations. You have reduced the risk of some very nasty diseases. It would be nice to promise you that you can now forget about your blood pressure and think of it as a problem in your past. Unfortunately, once you have been diagnosed as having high blood pressure, you will never be able to forget about it completely. Medication doesn't "cure" high blood pressure, so you may need to keep on taking the medicine for life. Changes in lifstyle don't "cure" high blood pressure either. If you brought down your pressure by losing weight, cutting out the sodium, and exercising, that's great—but remember that the pressure will go up again unless you keep up your good new habits.

So here are some final words to live by:

- See your doctor as often as the doctor suggests you should.

- Get your pressure measured regularly, or do it yourself.

- If you are on medication, take it! Don't *ever* stop taking the medicine or reduce the dosage on your own—always work with your doctor in making changes to medications.

- Look on the bright side. Your problem has been diagnosed in time. High blood pressure *can* be treated, preventing all the dangerous problems it can cause.

- And if you have made some of the changes suggested in this book, you are probably healthier all over as a result.

artery   Blood vessels that carry blood from the heart to different parts of the body. Arteries expand and contract slightly as blood flows through them.

atherosclerosis   Buildup in the arteries due to deposits of cholesterol and other substances. As the buildup increases, the arteries become narrowed and may be blocked completely (often because a blood clot gets stuck where the artery is narrow).

cholesterol   A fatlike substance ("lipid") found in all animal tissue. It's only present in food that comes from animals, including meat, fish, poultry, eggs, animal fats like lard, and dairy products. Excess cholesterol from the diet helps increase blood cholesterol levels, which can lead to blockage of the arteries.

coronary arteries   Tiny arteries (no more than about one-eighth inch across) that supply blood to the heart muscle itself. Heart attacks are caused when a coronary artery is blocked and the heart muscle is deprived of the oxygen carried by the blood.

diastolic blood pressure   The lower of the two measurements of blood pressure. It gives the pressure in the artery when the heart is relaxing between beats.

heart attack   Sudden interruption of blood flow to part of the heart muscle, resulting in its damage or death. Most heart attacks are caused by blockages in the coronary arteries which supply blood to the heart.

high blood pressure (or hypertension)   A chronic increase in blood pressure above its normal range.

high density lipoprotein (HDL)   The "good" type of cholesterol, which can transport the "bad" types away from the tissues.

hypertension   See "high blood pressure."

obesity   Being significantly overweight—usually, 30% or more above ideal body weight.

potassium   An important mineral in the body that is found mainly inside of cells. High levels of potassium in the diet help to maintain normal blood pressure levels.

saturated fats   Types of dietary fat that are "saturated" with hydrogen, and that help raise levels of cholesterol in the blood. These fats are found mainly in foods of animal origin, and a few of plant origin, such as tropical oils. Saturated fats are usually solid at room temperature.

sodium   A mineral that is found in nearly all plant and animal tissue. Excess sodium in the diet can raise blood pressure, and make it hard to bring down. Table salt (sodium chloride) is nearly half sodium.

stethoscope   Listening instrument that is used to hear sounds of blood flowing through the artery as blood pressure is measured.

stroke   A sudden shortage of blood in the brain, caused when the blood supply is interrupted by the blockage of an artery or when an artery bursts.

systolic blood pressure   The higher of the two blood pressure measurements, showing the pressure within the artery while the heart is contracting.

Suggestions for Further Reading

Bailey, C. 1991. *The New Fit or Fat.* New York: Houghton Mifflin.

Brody, Jane. 1987. *The Good Food Book.* New York: Bantam.

Connor, S. and W. Connor. 1983. *The New American Diet System.* New York: Simon and Schuster.

Farquhar, J. 1987. *The American Way of Life Need Not Be Hazardous to Your Health.* Reading: Addison Wesley.

Krauss, B. 1990. *The Dictionary of Sodium, Fats & Cholesterol.* Berkeley: Berkeley Publishers.

Robertson, L. 1986. *The New Laurel's Kitchen.* Berkeley: Ten Speed Press.

Roth, H. 1983. *Deliciously Low.* New York: New American Library.

——— 1986. *Deliciously Simple.* New York: New American Library.

Starke, Rodman and Mary Winston. 1990. *The American Heart Association Low-Salt Cookbook.* New York: Times Books.

Warshaw, H. S. 1993. *Eat Out, Eat Right.* Chicago: Surrey Books.

——— 1990. *The Restaurant Companion.* Chicago: Surrey Books.

Williams, J. 1986. *Quick and Delicious Low-Fat, Low-Salt Cookbook.* New York: Pedigree Books.